TALKING TO THE PSYCHIATRIST

BIPOLARITY

AF797499

Editing: Randy Saborit Mora
Proofreading: Randy Saborit Mora
Interior design and layout: Danayris Caballero García
Cover design: Otane González Martínez

La Fe Medical Clinic: medical services and publication of educational and self-help books on mental health and general medicine topics, with a human and accessible approach. For more information on how to obtain copies or access other resources on emotional health or medical services, visit our websites:

La Fe Medical Clinic
3030 East 4th Street
Los Ángeles, CA 90063
www.lafeclinic.com
www.telegalenos.com
www.miamigodoctor.com

The book *Talking to the Psychiatrist: Bipolarity* is part of the *Telegalenos a gabacha quitá collection*, created to offer clear, compassionate, and science-based guidance to those facing mental or emotional health challenges. With warm, respectful, and accessible language, Dr. Alexis Gómez González, clinical psy- chiatrist, accompanies the reader with empathy, experience, and knowledge.

Talking to the Psychiatrist: Bipolarity
Written by Dr. Alexis Gómez González
ISBN: 978-1-968561-20-8

TALKING TO THE PSYCHIATRIST

BIPOLARITY

ALEXIS GÓMEZ GONZÁLEZ

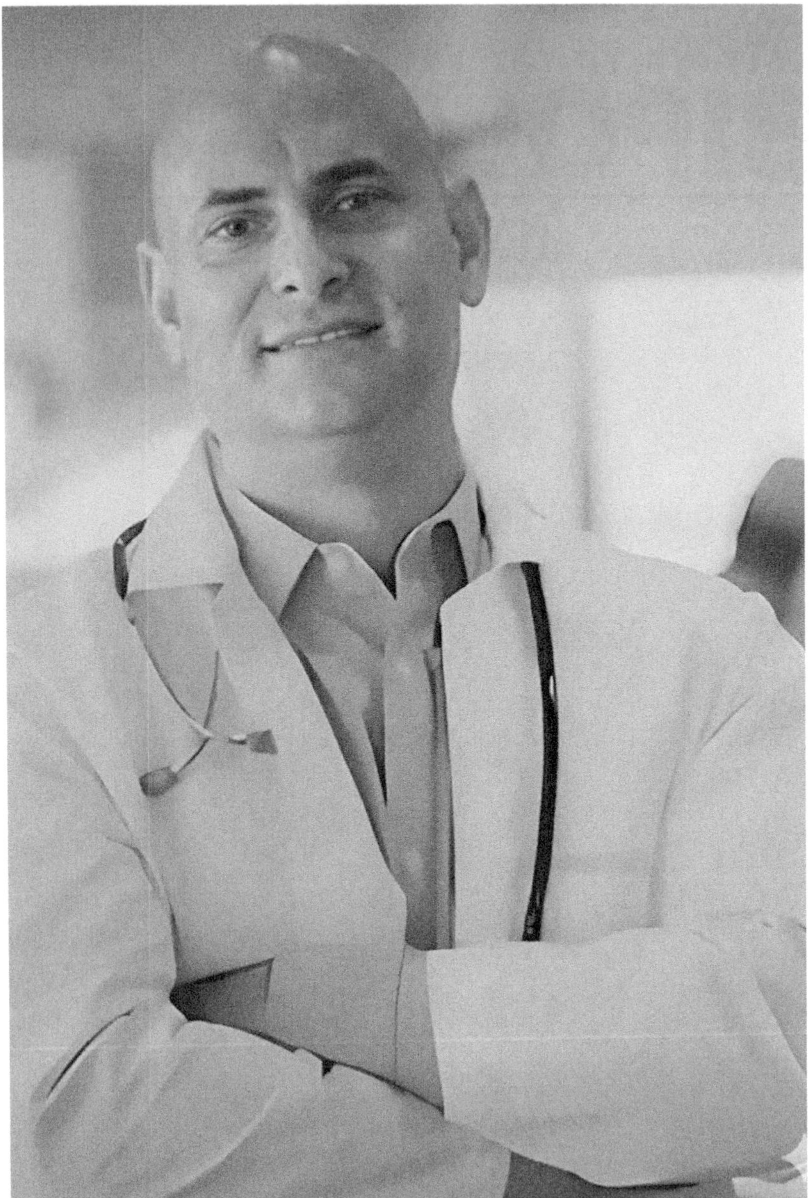

Author Introduction

My name is Alexis Gómez González. I am a medical graduate of the School of Medical Sciences in Havana and the University of Long Beach, California, with a specialty and master's degree in family medicine and psychiatry. In my more than 26 years of clinical, community and teaching experience, I have worked in areas of family medicine and psychiatry in communities in Cuba, Mexico and the United States, dedicating his career to humanizing medicine and bringing it closer to those who need it most.

I have dedicated my career to the comprehensive care of mental disorders, with special emphasis on anxiety, depression, insomnia, addictions and neurodevelopmental disorders. Trained in medicine and psychiatry, I have combined clinical knowledge with a passion for teaching and accessible outreach. I have created innovative graphic materials, helped patients, families, and healthcare professionals clearly and empathetically understand the complexity of the human mind, and worked on creating an approach that integrates science, compassion, and visual language as therapeutic and educational tools.

I currently run a clinic in Los Angeles and another in Mexico City, focused on the humanistic and effective treatment of psychiatric problems, especially in vulnerable populations. I also participate in medical training projects, creation of illustrated books and community care.

Acknowledgements

This book would not have been possible without the support and contribution of many people. We are deeply grateful to the mental health professionals, researchers, and experts who have shared their knowledge and experiences to enrich the content of this text.

Special thanks to the patients and their families, who have allowed their stories to be part of this work, which has allowed us to provide an invaluable perspective on the experience of bipolarity.

To our editor and our collaborators, whose effort and dedication have made the publication of this book possible. Their support has been critical at every stage of the process.

Finally, we thank all readers who seek to understand and overcome bipolarity. Their commitment to learning and growth is inspiring and essential to advancing mental health management.

Table of Contents

Introduction 35

PART I. Understanding Bipolar Disorder

CHAPTER 1 What Is Bipolar Disorder? An Introduction to the Oscillating Mind?

1.1 A Mind that Oscillates on Its Own Axes 41
1.2 A Clinical Definition, Various Human Realities 41
1.3 The First-Person Bipolar Experience 42
1.4 The Neurochemical Heart of Oscillation 42
1.5 A Common, but Often Invisible Condition 43
1.6 Bipolar Disorder in History and Culture 43
1.7 The Impact on Everyday Life 43
1.8 The Central Message 44

CHAPTER 2 History of Bipolar Disorder: from Greek Melancholy to Modern Stabilization

2.1 Greece and Rome: Melancholy and Mania as Poles of the Same Phenomenon 45
2.2 The Middle Ages and the Islamic World: between Demonology and Compassionate Hospitals 45

2.3 Renaissance and Enlightenment: from the "Evil of the Soul" to Moral Treatment 46
2.4 Nineteenth Century: Modern Diagnosis is Born 46
2.5 First Third of the Twentieth Century: Institutionalization and Shock Therapies 46
2.6 The Lithium Revolution 47
2.7 Antidepressants and the Recognition of Bipolar II 47
2.8 Atypical Anticonvulsants and Antipsychotics 47
2.9 From DSM-I to DSM-5: Specifying the Language 48
2.10 From Categorical to Dimensional Model: the "Bipolar Spectrum" 48
2.11 Human Rights, Destigmatization and Community 48
2.12 Timeline: Essential Milestones 48
2.13 Clinical Pearls and Historical Errors that we must not Repeat 49

CHAPTER 3 PHistorical and Artistic Characters with Bipolarity: between Genius and Chaos

3.1 Introduction 51
3.2 Vincent van Gogh. The Painter of the Turbulent Soul 51
3.3 Virginia Woolf. The Voice that Listened to the Tides of the Mind 51
3.4 Sylvia Plath. Poetry as a Scalpel of the Soul 52
3.5 Kanye West. Hypermodernity and Real-Time Mania 52
3.6 Carrie Fisher. Humor as a Lifesaver 52
3.7 Conclusions 53

CHAPTER 4 Depictions in Film, Literature and Musica

4.1 The Power of Art to Make Bipolarity Visible 55
4.2 Bipolarity in Cinema: Realism, Drama and Stigma 55
4.2.1 Science and Myth in Cinema 56

4.3 Literature: the Inner Voice of Bipolar Disorder 56
4.4 Music: Rhythm, Emotion and Bipolarity 56
4.5 Impact on Social Perception and Current Challenges 57
4.6 What to Learn from these Representations? 57
4.7 Conclusion 58

CHAPTER 5 Types of Bipolar Disorder: Bipolar I, II, Cyclothymia and Intermediate Spectra

5.1 The Diversity of the Same Fire 59
5.2 Bipolar Disorder Type I. The Summit of Lightning 59
5.3 Bipolar Disorder Type II. The Silent Fire 60
5.4 The Emotional Paradox 61
5.5 Cyclothymia. The Subtle Swing 61
5.6 Mixed Forms and Fast Cycles. When the Soul Runs and Cries at the Same Time 62
5.7 Art, Literature and the Types of Bipolarity 63
5.8 The Family and Social Perspective 64
5.9 The Map of Bipolarity 64

CHAPTER 6 Common Myths and Common Diagnostic Errors

6.1 When the Myth Disguises itself as Truth 67
6.2 Myth 1: "We're all a Little Bipolar" 67
6.3 Myth 2: "Bipolar People are Dangerous" 68
6.4 Myth 3: "Drugs Turn off Personality" 68
6.5 Myth 4: "Bipolar Disorder is Cured with Willpower" 68
6.6 Myth 5: "Bipolar is just a Form of Depression" 69
6.7 Common Clinical Error: Confusing Bipolar with ADHD or Borderline 69
6.8 Common Clinical Error: Underestimating the Role of Sleep and Hormones 69
6.9 The Impact of Stigma 70

6.10 Re-educating the Gaze 70
6.11 Final Recommendations for Professionals 70
6.12 Conclusion 70

PART II. Neurobiological and Neurochemical bases

CHAPTER 7 The Bipolar Brain: Regions Involved in Mania and Depression

7.1 The Internal Mood Scenario 75
7.2 The Emotional Brain: The Symphony of the Limbic System 75
7.3 The Prefrontal Cortex: The Regulator of Judgment 76
7.4 The Basal Ganglia and the Reward Circuit 76
7.5 The HPA Axis and Chronic Stress 77
7.6 Neural Networks Involved 77
7.7 Neuroimaging: the Visual Signature of Bipolar Disorder 77
7.8 Cerebral Laterality and Bipolar Creativity 78
7.9 Brain Plasticity and Therapeutic Hope 78
7.10 The Inner Dance 78

CHAPTER 8 Key Neurotransmitters: Dopamine, Serotonin, Glutamate, GABA, Norepinephrine and more

8.1 The Chemistry that Thinks us 81
8.2 Dopamine. The Fuel of Euphoria and Creativity 81
8.3 Serotonin. The Architect of Emotional Balance 82
8.4 Noradrenaline. The Energy of the Alert 82
8.5 GABA. The Brain Brake 83
8.6 Glutamato. The Spark of Arousal 83
8.7 Other Couriers Involved 83
8.8 Interactions and Balance 84
8.9 Integrative Example 84
8.10 Modern Therapeutic Perspective 85
8.11 The Messengers of the Soul 86

CHAPTER 9 Circadian Rhythm, Sleep-Wake Cycle and Seasonal Dysregulation

9.1 The Biological Clock of the Soul 87
9.2 Circadian Rhythm and Mood 87
9.3 Sleep: The Bipolar Balance Thermometer 87
9.4 Melatonin and Light: the Guardians of the Internal Clock 88
9.5 Hormonal Rhythms and Seasons of the Year 88
9.6 Chronotherapy and Sleep-Wake Regulation 89
9.7 Interaction between Sleep, Neurotransmitters and Episodes 89
9.8 Evolutionary and Social Perspective 89
9.9 Prevention and Self-Care 90
9.10 Synchronizing the Mind with Time 91

CHAPTER 10 Inflammation, Neuroplasticity and Mitochondrial Dysfunction in Bipolar Disorder

10.1 The Brain as a Biological Field 93
10.2 Inflammation as a Silent Root 93
10.3 Clinical Example 93
10.4 Microglia: The Inflammatory Guardians of the Brain 94
10.5 Neuroplasticity: the Power to Reinvent Yourself 94
10.6 Mitochondria: The Mood Energy Factories 95
10.7 Oxidation, Stress and Neuronal Aging 95
10.8 The Mind-Body Connection: Emotional Inflammation 95
10.9 Therapeutic and Scientific Perspective 96
10.10 The Fire That Heals 97

CHAPTER 11 PDNP-21-B Profile: Neurochemical Assessment of Bipolar

11.1 The Neurochemical Signature of Bipolar Disorder 99
11.2 The Principle of the DNP-21 Model 99
11.3 The Three Neurochemical Faces of Bipolar 100

11.4 Clinical Interpreting 101
11.5 Integrative Clinical Example 101
11.6 Clinical and Research Applications 102
11.7 Limitations and Future Projection 102
11.8 The Mapping of the Mood 103

PART III. Clinical Phases and Symptoms

CHAPTER 12 Manic Phase: Euphoria, Impulsivity, Hypersexuality and Delusions

12.1 The Rise of the Storm 107
12.2 The Early Signs 107
12.3 Manic Euphoria 107
12.4 Impulsivity and Loss of Judgment 108
12.5 Hypersexuality and Overflowing Desire 108
12.6 Verbiage and Racing Thinking 109
12.7 Irritability and Aggressiveness 109
12.8 Delusions and Psychotic Symptoms 109
12.9 Neurobiology of Mania 110
12.10 Consequences and Cumulative Damage 110
12.11 Therapeutic Strategy 110
12.12 The Light That Blinds 111

CHAPTER 13 Depressive Phase: Hopelessness, Mental Slowness and Suicidal Risk

13.1 The Silent Descent 113
13.2 The Slowness of Thought 113
13.3 Anhedonia: Offline Pleasure 113
13.4 Fatigue, Sleep and Altered Circadian Rhythm 114
13.5 Guilt, Self-Criticism and Hopelessness 114
13.6 Suicidal Risk 114

13.7 The Depressive Body 115
13.8 Differences with Unipolar Depression 115
13.9 Therapeutic Strategies 116
13.10 The Winter of the Mind 116

CHAPTER 14 Mixed Episodes: when the Body Runs but the Soul Cries

14.1 Two Storms in the Same Sky 119
14.2 What Happens in the Brain during a Mixed Episode? 119
14.3 Typical Symptoms of the Mixed Episode 120
14.5 The Highest Risk: Hopeless Energy 121
14.6 Differential Diagnosis 121
14.7 Therapeutic Management 121
14.8 Subjective Experience 122
14.9 Recovery and Follow-up 122
14.10 Lightning and Shadow 123

CHAPTER 15 Hypomania: Energy Disguised as Success

15.1 The Most Deceptive Phase of Bipolar Disorder 125
15.2 The Functional Face of Hypomania 125
15.3 Neurobiology of Hypomania 125
15.4 Differences between Hypomania and Mania 126
15.5 The Risk of False Well-Being 127
15.6 Creative Hypomania versus Destructive Hypomania 127
15.7 Clinical Approach 127
15.8 Hypomania in Art and Science 128
15.9 The Mirage of Equilibrium 128

CHAPTER 16 Psychotic Symptoms in Extreme Phases

16.1 The Mind That Overflows Reality 129
16.2 The Boundary Between Emotion and Perception 129
16.3 Types of Psychotic Symptoms in Bipolar Disorder 129

16.4 Neurobiology of Bipolar Psychosis 131
16.5 Treatment 131
16.6 Differences with Schizophrenia 132
16.7 Humanistic Perspective 132
16.8 The Mind that Saw Too Much 133

PART IV. Diagnosis and Evaluation

CHAPTER 17 Psychiatric Interview Focused on the Bipolar Spectrum

17.1 Diagnosing Movement, Not Timing 137
17.2 The Importance of the Vital Context 137
17.3 Clinical Dialogue 137
17.4 Phases as Emotional Language 138
17.5 Behavioral and Nonverbal Observation 139
17.6 Use of DNP-21-B as an Integrative Tool 139
17.7 Suicidal and Functional Risk Assessment 139
17.8 Common Diagnostic Difficulties 140
17.9 The Art of Rapport 141
17.10 Diagnosing with Empathy and Science 141

CHAPTER 18 DNP-21-B Diagnostic Scales and Neurochemical Profile

18.1 When Emotion Translates into Numbers 143
18.2 Measuring Euphoria 143
18.3 Detecting the Hidden Spectrum 144
18.4 Functional Brightness 144
18.5 The Clinician's Gaze 145
18.6 The Neurochemical Map of the Bipolar Spectrum 145
18.7 Practical Integration 146
18.8 Science that Listens 148

CHAPTER 19 Differential Diagnosis: ADHD, Borderline, Schizophrenia and Unipolar Depression
19.1 Bipolarity in Disguise 149
19.2 Bipolar Disorder versus Unipolar Depression 149
19.3 Bipolar Disorder versus ADHD 150
19.4 Bipolar Disorder versus Borderline Personality Disorder 151
19.5 Bipolar Disorder versus Schizophrenia 152
19.6 Other Common Confusions 153
19.7 The DNP-21-B as a Differentiation Tool 153
19.8 Diagnose with Accuracy and Compassion 154
CHAPTER 20 Bipolar Disorder in Children, Adolescents and Older Adults
20.1 Same Storm, Different Ages 157
20.2 Bipolar Disorder in Childhood. The Energy that the Brain cannot yet Tame 157
20.3 Bipolar Disorder in Adolescence. The Brain in Metamorphosis 158
20.4 Bipolar Disorder in Adulthood. The Possible Balance 159
20.5 Bipolar Disorder in the Elderly. The Storm under the Calm 159
20.6 Neuroevolutionary Approach. The Dopamine Cycle and Emotional Wisdom 160
20.7 The Same Melody in Different Keys 161
CHAPTER 21 Most Common Errors in Diagnosing Bipolar Disorder
21.1 The Cost of Late Diagnosis 163
21.2 Mistake 1: Confusing Bipolar with Unipolar Depression 163
21.3 Mistake 2: Labeling as ADHD what is Juvenile Bipolar 164
21.4 Mistake 3: Confusing with Borderline 164
21.5 Mistake 4: Ignoring the Biological and Neurochemical Component 164

21.6 Mistake 5: Diagnosing Generalized Anxiety 165
21.7 Mistake 6: Believing that the Patient Exaggerates 165
21.8 Mistake 7: Not Educating the Patient or Family 165
21.9 DNP-21-B as an Antidote to Diagnostic Error 166
21.10 Diagnose with Humility and Depth 167

PART V. Pharmacological Treatment

CHAPTER 22 Mood Stabilizers: Lithium, Valproate, Lamotrigine and Carbamazepine

22.1 The Chemistry of Stability 171
22.2 Lithium, the Element of Balance 171
22.3 Valproate. The Shield of Inhibition 172
22.4 Lamotrigine. The Light and Shadow Stabilizer 173
22.5 Carbamazepine. The Guardian of Neuronal Fire 174
22.6 Choosing the Right Stabilizer 174
22.7 Integrative and Future Perspectives 175
22.8 The Science of Balance 175

CHAPTER 23 Atypical Antipsychotics: Quetiapine, Olanzapine, Lurasidone and Aripiprazole

23.1 When Excess Dopamine Turns to Noise 177
23.2 Quetiapine: the Inner Storm Soothing 177
23.3 Olanzapine: the Energy Stabilizer 178
23.4 Lurasidone: Clarity without Sedation 178
23.5 Aripiprazole: the Dopaminergic System Modulator 179
23.6 DNP-21-B Selection 180
23.7 Beyond the Stigma 180
23.8 The Art of Modulating Dopamine 181

CHAPTER 24 Cautious Use of Antidepressants in Bipolar Disorder

24.1 The Double-Edged Serotonin 183
24.2 Neurochemical Basis: Serotonin, Dopamine, and the Oscillation Axis 183
24.3 Types of Antidepressants and Risk of Swerving 184
24.4 The Golden Rule: Never in Monotherapy 184
24.5 Early Signs of Manic Turning 185
24.6 Strategies for the Prudent Use of Antidepressants 185
24.7 Non-Antidepressant Alternatives for the Bipolar Depressive 186
24.8 Special Considerations 186
24.9 Pharmacological Humility 187

CHAPTER 25 Benzodiazepines, Melatonin and Insomnia Management Associated with Bipolar Disorder

25.1 Sleep as a Natural Mood Stabilizer 189
25.2 Neurobiology of Sleep and Bipolarity 189
25.3 Benzodiazepines. The Nervous System's Brief Respite 190
25.4 Melatonin. The Molecular Clock of Mood 190
25.5 Non-Pharmacological Strategies for Bipolar Insomnia 191
25.6 Natural Alternatives and Emerging Therapies 191
25.7 Insomnia as a Sentinel Symptom 191
25.8 Sleep as a Form of Treatment 192

CHAPTER 26 New Biologic Therapies: Ketamine, Esketamine, Psilocybin, ECT and TMS

26.1 From Classical Pharmacology to the Synaptic Revolution 193
26.2 Ketamine, the Switch of Hopelessness 193
26.3 Esketamine, the Controlled Evolution of Ketamine 194
26.4 Psilocybin, the Science-Based inner Journey 194
26.5 ECT: Electrical Therapy that Saved Thousands of Minds 195
26.6 TMS, Transcranial Magnetic Stimulation 195

26.7 Neuroplasticity and Integrative Psychotherapy 196
26.8 Science, Mysticism and Hope 196

CHAPTER 27 EKG Monitoring, Plasma Levels and Long-Term Security

27.1 To Treat is also to Care 197
27.2 The Heart as a Mirror of Neurochemical Balance 197
27.3 Monitoring of Plasma Levels 198
27.4 Metabolism and Weight Control. The Silent Enemy 199
27.5 Renal, Hepatic and Thyroid Evaluation 199
27.6 Long-Term Security. Beyond Chemistry 200
27.7 Integration of Monitoring into the DNP-21-B Model 200
27.8 The Medicine of Observation 201

CHAPTER 28 Clinical Algorithms per Phase: Acute Mania, Bipolar Maintenance and Depression

28.1 Psychiatry as Dynamic Cartography 203
28.2 Acute manic phase 203
28.3 Bipolar Depressive Phase 204
28.4 Mixed Phase 205
28.5 Maintenance Phase 206
28.6 DNP-21-B Integrative Algorithm 207
28.7 Chaos at the Algorithm 208

PART VI. Non-Pharmacological Interventions

CHAPTER 29 Cognitive-Behavioral Therapy Adapted to Bipolarity

29.1 The Mind as a Laboratory of Change 211
29.2 Neurocognitive Basis of Bipolar Thinking 211
29.3 Core Tools of Adapted CBT 212
29.4 Clinical Example 212

29.5 Integration of CBT with Other Therapies 214
29.6 Thinking with Tenderness and Discipline 214
CHAPTER 30 Individual and Family Psychoeducation
30.1 Educating to Stabilize 215
30.2 Objectives of Bipolar Psychoeducation 216
30.3 Individual Psychoeducation 216
30.4 Family Psychoeducation. Allies Instead of Judges 217
30.5 The DNP-21-B Model Applied to Psychoeducation 217
30.6 Group Dynamics and Educational Resources 218
30.7 Knowing is Caring 218
CHAPTER 31 Interpersonal and Social Rhythm Therapy
31.1 Time as Medicine 219
31.2 Biological and Emotional Foundations of Social Rhythm 219
31.3 Structure of the IPSRT 220
31.4 Neurochemical Intervention 220
31.5 Clinical Example 221
31.6 IPSRT as a Bridge between Science and Everyday Life 222
31.7 The Melody of Inner Time 222
CHAPTER 32 Acceptance and Commitment Therapy and DBTT
32.1 From Control to Conscious Acceptance 223
32.2 Acceptance and Commitment Therapy (ACT) 223
32.3 Dialectical Behavioural Therapy (DBT) 224
32.4 Neurobiology of Emotional Acceptance and Regulation 225
32.5 ACT + DBT Integration in Bipolar Treatment 225
32.6 Acceptance as an Inner Revolution 225
CHAPTER 33 Mindfulness, Meditation and Mind-Body Techniques
33.1 The Body as an Entrance to the Mind 227
33.2 Mindfulness: Full Attention without Judgment 227

33.3 Meditation: The Neuroscience of Silence 228
33.4 Body-Mind Techniques: Physiology of Stability 228
33.5 Integration with the DNP-21-B Model 230
33.6 Serenity as a Daily Practice 230

CHAPTER 34 Social Support, Psychoeducational Groups and Rehabilitation Programs

34.1 Stability as a Collective Construction 231
34.2 The Clinical Value of Social Support 231
34.3 Psychoeducational Groups. Learning in Community 232
34.4 Psychosocial Rehabilitation Programmes 232
34.5 Integration with the DNP-21-B 233
34.6 The Role of the Family and Community Environment 234
34.7 Healing in the Plural 234

PART VII. The Impact on Life

CHAPTER 35 Bipolar Disorder at Work, Studies and Professional Life

35.1 The Challenge of Functioning 237
35.2 Challenges of the Work and Academic Environment 237
35.3 Strategies for Job and Academic Stability 238
35.4 Reasonable Accommodations 238
35.5 Emotional Education in the Professional Field 238
35.6 DNP-21-B Model Applied to Professional Performance 239
35.7 Redefining Success 240

CHAPTER 36 Affective Relationships, Family and Emotional Conflict Management

36.1 Love as a Mirror of the Mind 241
36.2 How do Bipolar Phases Affect Relationships? 241
36.3 Conscious and Emotionally Safe Communication 242
36.4 Family: Allies, Not Judges 242
36.5 Sexuality and Intimate Ties 243

36.6 The DNP-21-B Model in Couple and Family Dynamics 244
36.7 Loving from Inner Stability 244

CHAPTER 37 Sexuality, Impulsivity and Self-Esteem

37.1 Desire in an Oscillating Brain 245
37.2 The Neurochemistry of Desire 245
37.3 Hypersexuality and Behavioral Risk 246
37.4 Depression, Body and Self-Esteem 247
37.5 Self-Esteem and Conscious Sexuality 248
37.6 Integration with the DNP-21-B Model 248
37.7 The Reconciled Body 249

CHAPTER 38 Bipolar Disorder and Addictions: Common Comorbidities

38.1 Two Disorders That Are Enhanced 251
38.2 Why is the Bipolar Brain more Vulnerable to Addictions? 251
38.3 Substances most Associated with Bipolar Disorder 252
38.4 Dual Diagnosis and Integrated Treatment 253
38.5 Recommended Therapeutic Strategies 253
38.6 Integration with the DNP-21-B Model 253
38.7 Regaining Control Without Losing Hope 255

CHAPTER 39 Suicide Risk: Assessment, Prevention and Accompaniment

39.1 Suicide as an Expression of Invisible Suffering 257
39.2 Neurobiology of Suicidal Drive 257
39.3 Risk Factors and Warning Signs 258
39.4 Clinical Assessment of Suicide Risk 258
39.5 Prevention and Management Strategies 259
39.6 The Role of Lithium and Neuroprotection 259
39.7 Integration with the DNP-21-B Model 260
39.8 Hope as a Treatment 260

CHAPTER 40 Crisis, Hospitalizations and Emergency Managements
40.1 The Crisis as a Turning Point 263
40.2 Early Identification of a Crisis 263
40.3 Clinical Evaluation During Emergency 264
40.4 Hospitalization: when and why? 265
40.5 Emergency Management at Home or Consultation 265
40.6 Emergency and Containment Drugs 266
40.7 Integration with the DNP-21-B Model 266
40.8 From Crisis to Growth 267

PART VIII. Integrative And Holistic Approaches

CHAPTER 41 Physical Exercise and Mental Health
41.1 The Body as a Natural Stabilizer of Mood 271
41.2 Neurochemical Effects of Exercise 271
41.3 Recommended Types of Exercise for Bipolar Patients 272
41.4 The Risk of Excess: Exercise and Mania 272
41.5 Integration of Exercise into the Therapeutic Plan 273
41.6 Movement as Medicine of the Soul 274

CHAPTER 42 Nutrition, Inflammation and Brain Microbiota
42.1 The New Frontier of Nutritional Psychiatry 275
42.2 Brain Inflammation and Dysfunction 275
42.3 The Gut Microbiota: an Ecosystem that Influences Mood 276
42.4 Nutrients that Protect the Bipolar Brain 277
42.5 The Inflammatory Model of Bipolar Disorder 277
42.6 Integration with the DNP-21-B 278
42.7 Eating as a Therapeutic Act 279

CHAPTER 43 Restful Sleep as a Cornerstone of Treatment
43.1 Sleep as a Neurochemical Regulator 281
43.2 Neurobiology of Sleep in the Bipolar Brain 281

43.3 Most Common Types of Sleep Disturbances 282
43.4 Sleep Deprivation as a Trigger for Relapse 282
43.5 Clinical Strategies for Restoring Sleep 283
43.6 Integration with the DNP-21-B Model 284
43.7 Rest as an Invisible Medicine 284
CHAPTER 44 Spirituality, Meaning of Life and Existential Crises
44.1 Beyond the Diagnosis: the Hunger for Meaning 285
44.2 Neurobiology of Spirituality 286
44.3 Existential Crisis 286
44.4 Spirituality and Resilience 286
44.5 Clinical Integration of the Spiritual Approach 287
44.6 Integration with the DNP-21-B 287
44.7 When the Mind Finds Its Purpose 288
CHAPTER 45 The Model of Medical Aikido Applied to Bipolarity (2A + 2B + 2C + 2D)
45.1 General Framework: Why "Aikido" in Mental Health? 289
45.2 Practical Neurobiology of the Model 289
45.3 The 2A with Measurable Protocols 291
45.3.1 Anticipating: Signal Map and Risk Window 291
45.3.2 Analyze: Trigger Matrix and Microadjustment Decisions 292
45.4 The 2B with Guided Exercises 292
45.4.1 Welcome: 90-second Interoceptive Exposure 292
45.4.2 Benevolence: Micro-self-compassion with Prosody 292
45.5 The 2C with Power Transfer Tools 293
45.5.1 Control: 6-stop Kit of 60-120 Seconds 293
45.5.2 Change: Behavioral Substitution and Creative Channel 293
45.6 The 2D with Science of Thought and Closure 294
45.6.1 Tear Down: Belief Therapy with Behavioral Experiments 294

45.6.2 Dissolving: Neurobiological Closure Practices 294
45.7 Differential Protocols by Phase 295
45.7.1 Hypomania/Mania Protocol (24-72 h) 295
45.7.2 Bipolar Depression Protocol (7-14 days) 295
45.8 DNP-21-B Integration: Custom Prescribing 296
45.9 Working with Family and Couple: Relational Aikido 297
45.10 Weekly Practice Plan (30 days, renewable) 297
45.11 Measurement-Based Care 297
45.12 Motivating Ending Vignettes 298
45.13 Transforming Practice 299

PART IX. Recovery and Resilience

CHAPTER 46 What Does This Remission Mean?

46.1 Remission Does not Mean Definitive Cure 303
46.2 Types of Remission: Clinical, Syndromic and Functional 303
46.3 Stabilization Does not Mean Cure 303
46.4 Practical Criteria for Sustained Remission 304
46.5 How Do We Measure Remission?: Minimum Follow-up 304
46.6 Summary Neurobiology of Remission 305
46.7 Residuals that Matter: Small Symptoms, Big Risks 305
46.8 Recommended Maintenance Duration After Referral 305
46.9 Therapeutic Principles in Remission 306
46.10 Early Signs and Rapid Action Plan 306
46.11 Brief Clinical Maintenance Algorithm 307
46.12 Patient Education: How to Explain It in Consultation? 307
46.13 Referral Checklist for the control Visit 307
46.14 Weekly Self-Monitoring Sheet (Suggested Format) 307
46.15 Conclusion 308

CHAPTER 47 Life Projects with Bipolarity: Realism and Hope

47.1 Lucid Stability: the Alchemy between Biology and Purpose 309
47.2 Therapeutic Realism: the Wisdom of the Midpoint 309

47.3 Redefining Success 310
47.4 Axes of the Stable Life Project 310
47.5 Neurobiology of Hope 311
47.6 Therapies of Meaning and Reinvention 311
47.7 Clinical Example 312
47.8 Practical Strategies 312
47.9 The Environment as a Regulatory System 312
47.10 From Ideal Sleep to Sustainable Purpose 313

CHAPTER 48 Doctor-patient Relationship

48.1 Enduring Therapeutic Alliance 315
48.2 The neurobiology of the therapeutic link 315
48.3 Phases of the Alliance in the Bipolar Patient 316
48.4 Clinical Empathy and Professional Boundaries 316
48.5 Effective Therapeutic Communication 316
48.6 Confidence, Adherence and Prognosis 317
48.7 The Doctor as a Regulating Mirror 317
48.8 The Patient as the Protagonist 317
48.9 Critical Moments: Rupture and Repair 318
48.10 Telemedicine and Digital Humanity 318
48.11 Existential Alliance 318

CHAPTER 49 Relapse Prevention: Early Signs and Action Plans

49.1 Introduction 321
49.2 Understanding the Neurobiological Terrain of Risk 321
49.3 The Three Phases of Relapse 322
49.4 Specific Early Signs 322
49.5 The 10 Strongest Predictors of Relapse 323
49.6 Neuropsychoeducation: Teaching How to Read the Signs 323
49.7 Construction of the Personal Prevention Plan 323
49.8 The Role of the Environment 324
49.9 Technology and Prevention 324
49.10 Psychology of Prevention 325

49.11 Psychiatric Emergencies and First Aid 325
49.12 Conclusions 325

CHAPTER 50 Recovery Stories: Patients Who Inspire
50.1 Introduction 327
50.2 Laura, the Architect of Rhythm 327
50.3 Andrew, the Mentor of the Second Chance 328
50.4 Diana, the Artist Who Painted Her Balance 328
50.5 Samuel, the Body as Medicine 329
50.6 Mariana, the Scientist Mother 329
50.7 Daniel, the Philosopher of Inner Balance 330
50.8 Conclusions 330

PART X. Treatment According Population Group

CHAPTER 51 Bipolar in Women: Hormonal Cycle, Pregnancy and Postpartum
51.1 Introduction 335
51.2 Menstrual Cycle 335
51.3 Pregnancy 336
51.4 Postpartum 336
51.5 Menopause 338
51.6 Conclusions 338

CHAPTER 52 Childhood and Adolescent Bipolarity: Early Diagnoses and Controversies
52.1 Introduction 341
52.2 Childhood 341
52.3 Adolescence 343
52.4 Psychoeducation for Parents 344
52.5 Conclusions 344

CHAPTER 53 Bipolar Disorder in Older Age: Medical Complications and Cognition
53.1 Bipolarity that Ages 347
53.2 Geriatric Bipolarity 347

53.3 Neurobiological Dimension: When Mood Slows Down 347
53.4 Medical Dimension: Comorbidities and Pharmacological Fragility 348
53.5 Cognitive Dimension: Affective Deterioration Without Loss of Humanity 348
53.6 Therapeutic Principles in the Elderly 349
53.7 The Environment and Attachments as Neurobiological Stabilizers 349
53.8 Cumulative Grief and Meaning Therapy 350
53.9 Spirituality and Lucid Serenity in Old Age 350
53.10 Late Neuroplasticity and Peace Learning 350
53.11 Emotional Wisdom and Mature Resilience 350
53.12 The Clinic as a Testimony of Life 351
53.13 Old Age as a Chapter of Psychiatric Wisdom 351

CHAPTER 54 Bipolar disorder with ADHD, Anxiety, Trauma, or Autism Spectrum

54.1 Introduction 353
54.2 Bipolarity and ADHD: Energy without Focus 353
54.3 Bipolarity and Anxiety: the Alarm System on Fire 354
54.4 Bipolarity and Trauma: the Memory that Does not Sleep 354
54.5 Bipolarity and the Autism Spectrum: Two Different Ways of Feeling the World 355
54.6 The Polyphonic Mind 355
54.7 Conclusions 356

PARTE XI. Where to Go for Help?

CHAPTER 55 Mexico: psychiatric hospitals, NGO, Digital platforms and crisis lines

55.1 Seeking Help as an Act of Clinical and Human Wisdom 359
55.2 National Mental Health System: Public Care Structure 359
55.3 Psychiatric Hospitals and National Referral Institutions 359
55.4 CISAME and Decentralized Community Care 360

55.5 Digital Platforms and Telepsychiatry in Mexico 360
55.6 Crisis Lines and Immediate Attention 361
55.7 NGO and Civil Associations: Support Beyond the System 361
55.8 Family, Community and Culture as Protective Factors 362
55.9 Towards a More Humane and Accessible Mental Health 362

CHAPTER 56 Spain: Public Services, Support Associations and Community Centers

56.1 Spain and the Community Model of Mental Health 363
56.2 National Health System: Public Access and Continuity of Care 363
56.3 Hospitals and Referral Centres for Bipolar Disorder 363
56.4 Day Centres 364
56.5 Patient and Family Associations: Accompaniment and Psychoeducation 364
56.6 The Family as an Active Therapeutic Agent 365
56.7 Digital Platforms and Emotional Support Lines 365
56.8 Crisis Care: Mobile Teams and Rapid Response 365
56.9 The Three Pillars of the Spanish Community Model 366
56.10 Precision Research and Psychiatry 366
56.11 Culture, Community and Dignity of Care 367
56.12 Mental Health as Shared Well-being 367

CHAPTER 57 United States: Community Clinics, Bilingual Resources & Emergency Services

57.1 Introduction 369
57.2 Community Mental Health Clinics 369
57.3 Bilingual Resources and Support for Immigrants 370
57.4 Crisis and Emergency Services 371
57.5 Education, Peer Networks, and Patient Advocacy 372
57.6 Challenges and Hope 372

PART XII. Psychic Energy in Motion

CHAPTER 58 Table of Neurotransmitters and Associated Bipolar Symptoms

58.1 The Bipolar Brain: Balance and Deregulation 377
58.2 Neurochemical Balance as a Therapeutic Art 379

CHAPTER 59 Emotional and Neurocognitive Map of Bipolar Disorder

59.1 The Brain as an Emotional Territory 381
59.2 Brain Networks: a Desynchronized Symphony 382
59.3 The Emotional Map: from Euphoria to Emptiness 382
59.4 The Cognitive Dimension: Thinking, Memory and Judgment 383
59.5 Consciousness as an Integrating Network 384
59.6 The Future: Neurocircuits of Hope 384

CHAPTER 60 Symbolic Gallery of Bipolar Disorder: Painting, Poetry and Cinema

60.1 Painting: Emotion Made Color 387
60.1.1 Vincent van Gogh, the Brush of the Inner Storm 387
60.1.2 Frida Kahlo, the Body as a Mirror of the Soul 387
60.1.3 Edvard Munch, the Cry of Imbalance 388
60.2 Poetry: The Alchemy of Emotion 388
60.2.1 Sylvia Plath, the Language of the Abyss 388
61.2.2 Federico García Lorca, the Luminous Tragedy 389
61.2.3 Anne Sexton, confession as catharsis 389
61.3 Cinema: the Narrative mirror of the Bipolar Mind 390
61.3.1 *A Beautiful Mind* (2001): The Genius and His Labyrinth 390
61.3.2 *Silver Linings Playbook* (2012): Love, Chaos and Neurochemistry 390
61.3.3 *The Hours* (2002): Three Women, one Abyss 391
61.4 Art as Therapy, Art as a Mirror 391
61.5 Towards an Aesthetics of Stability 391

CHAPTER 61 Model B-DNP-21 Applied to Bipolarity
61.1 What is the DNP-21 form? 393
61.2 Instrument B-DNP-21–Bipolar Disorder 394
61.3 Objective of questionnaire B-DNP-21 394
61.4 DNP-21 Questionnaire–Bipolar Disorder 396

Epilogue
Science as a Bridge to Compassion 401

Annotated Scientific Bibliography
Biological and Neurochemical Foundations 403
Psychotherapy and Integrative Approaches 404
Cultural and Existential Perspectives 405
Innovations, Neuroscience and the Future 405

Appendices
Appendix 1.
Digital, Educational, and Community Resources 407
Appendix 2.
100 Frequently Asked Questions in my Consultation 408

Therapeutic-emotional Glossary 419

***Telegalenos a gabacha quitá* Collection** 423

Foreword

Between the overflowing light and the deep shadow, it is necessary to understand bipolar disorder with science, compassion and humanity. It is not a simple mood swing but a profound medical condition that alters the rhythms of thought, sleep, energy and emotions, affecting the way a person lives, loves, works and dreams. It can transform euphoria into chaos and sadness into paralysis. But also, when it is understood and treated sensitively, it can open paths of self-knowledge, creativity and unsuspected resilience.

This book is born from the daily encounter between the psychiatrist and the patient, in that intimate space where one seeks to understand what the mind silences, what the body expresses, what the personal history drags along. It is part of the *Telegalenos a gabacha quitá* collection in which topics such as depression, anxiety, insomnia, dementia and schizophrenia have already been addressed, always from an integrative approach: scientific, human, clinical, symbolic, rigorous and compassionate.

Here we are not only talking about diagnoses and medicines. We are talking about neurotransmitters and circadian rhythms; but also of art, history, literature, spirituality, of broken and rebuilt ties. We dwell on figures such as Vincent van Gogh, Virginia Woolf or Kanye West, not out of morbidity, but to understand how bipolarity has inhabited --and transformed– great minds throughout history.

Through these pages you will find clear explanations about the types of bipolar disorder. Its causes, its neurochemistry, the available treatments (pharmacological and non-pharmacological), as well as therapeutic strategies applicable both in consultation and in daily life. Tools are also offered for family members, caregivers and health professionals who accompany this complex journey.

We also address the social and cultural dimension of diagnosis, stigma, excessive medicalization or denial of suffering, and how to build paths to recovery beyond pharmacological stabilization.

Because living with bipolarity does not mean living without direction. It means learning to navigate, with help, the inner tides. And this book is an open, informed, and respectful conversation. It does not intend to give unique answers, but to offer a map. An emotional, neurochemical and therapeutic map so that patients, families and professionals can make informed, compassionate and effective decisions.

If you've ever felt like a prisoner of your ups and downs, if you're accompanying someone who oscillates between hyperactivity and hopelessness, or if you're a mental health professional looking for gain a deeper understanding of this complex and fascinating disorder, this book is for you.

Welcome to this journey between mania and melancholy. Between neuroscience and poetry. Between chaos and the possibility of rebuilding.

Dr. Alexis Gómez González

Introduction

This treatise is aimed at psychiatrists, doctors, psychologists, nurses, patients with bipolar disorder and their families. It aims to be one of the most complete compendiums written on the subject, with a clinical, human, cultural and spiritual perspective.

It contains detailed explanations of neurotransmitter dynamics in mood regulation, the history of bipolar disorder over the centuries, differential diagnosis with other psychiatric conditions, pharmacological and non-pharmacological treatments, psychotherapies, lifestyle interventions, crisis prevention, and long-term recovery strategies. Throughout the text, he also offers a roadmap to understand bipolarity not only as a disorder, but as a profound challenge in mood regulation that implies suffering, but also growth potential.

Key contents of the book:

1. Medical, symbolic, and cultural definitions of bipolar disorder.
2. History of bipolarity in psychiatry: from "madness" to mood stabilization.
3. The bipolar spectrum: type I, type II, cyclothymia, mixed states, rapid cycling.
4. Neurobiological basis: neurotransmitters, circadian rhythms and brain circuits.
5. Genetic, psychological, and environmental factors.

6. The manic phase: euphoria, grandiosity, impulsivity and loss of judgment.
7. The depressive phase: slowing down, hopelessness and isolation.
8. Mixed episodes: agitation with despair.
9. Comprehensive diagnosis and frequent clinical errors.
10. Pharmacological treatment: mood stabilizers, antipsychotics, antidepressants and emerging therapies.
11. Non-pharmacological interventions: psychotherapy, lifestyle habits and sleep regulation.
12. Medical Aikido applied to bipolar disorder.
13. Crisis management and relapse prevention plans.
14. Family and community support.
15. Bipolar disorder in art, literature, and cultural history.
16. International resources: Mexico, Spain and the United States.
17. Final manifesto for a psychiatry with a soul.

Why does understanding bipolar disorder matter?

Bipolar disorder is not just "mood swings". It is a complex, recurrent, and potentially disabling condition that can bring both extraordinary creativity and profound suffering. It's not just being "too happy" or "too sad". It is a dysregulation of mood, energy, and thought patterns that requires medical, psychological, and social attention.

Understanding bipolar disorder from a scientific and compassionate perspective is the first step to building stable and meaningful lives for those who suffer from it. This book is an invitation to replace prejudice with knowledge, to see beyond extremes, to accompany without judgment and to understand that stability is possible with the right treatment, support and self-awareness.

I've seen people recover from destructive manic episodes and rebuild their relationships. I've watched others manage their depression without getting lost in hopelessness. I have witnessed how families have gone from chaos to collaboration.

This is not a book of magical cures: it is a practical and humane guide. It is not a sermon: it is a necessary conversation. Because not all suffering is visible. And not all stability is achieved with medication alone.

It is written with science, but also with empathy. With protocols, but also with stories. With data, but also with the language of human experience. If you read these pages feeling like your mind is a storm, remember this: storms pass. And even in the most unstable sky... There are always horizons ahead.

PART I.
Understanding Bipolar Disorder

CHAPTER 1
What Is Bipolar Disorder?

Between the luminous euphoria and the densest shadow.

1.1 A Mind that Oscillates on Its Own Axes

Imagine living in a world where the emotional climate changes in ways that are as intense as they are unexpected. Days when the sun shines with an almost painful intensity and fills everything with energy, ideas and movement... and suddenly, like a sudden eclipse, the sky is covered and the light disappears, and leaves a gloom that covers everything.

That's the emotional territory of bipolar disorder: a medical and neurochemical condition that not only alters mood, but alters the very course of life. Bipolar disorder is not "being happy and sad". It is a profound alteration in the regulation of energy, thought, sleep, perception and behavior. It's a change in the way the brain adjusts its own activity levels, as if the emotional thermostat is broken and oscillates between the most intense heat and the most paralyzing cold.

1.2 A Clinical Definition, Various Human Realities

Medically, bipolar disorder is classified in the DSM-5 as a mood disorder characterized by manic, hypomanic, and depressive episodes, which may alternate or coexist.

There are several types:

- Bipolar I: episodes of complete mania, often followed or preceded by major depression.
- Bipolar II: episodes of hypomania and major depression, without full mania.
- Cyclothymia: Milder but persistent chronic mood swings, lasting at least two years.

- Other specified and unspecified: atypical forms, with mixed symptoms or rapid cycling (four or more episodes per year).

But beyond the diagnostic label, each person lives their own version of bipolarity. For some, mania is a burst of creativity and social connection; for others, a dangerous spiral of impulsivity and risk. Depression, on the other hand, can be a time of painful introspection or an abyss from which it is difficult to get out.

1.3 The First-Person Bipolar Experience

Someone who experiences a manic episode can describe it as "having an engine that never turns off", "feeling that everything is possible" or "being connected to the universe on a higher level". But that overflowing energy often comes at a cost: excessive spending of money, impulsive decisions, risky sexual behaviors, fights, loss of relationships, and, in extreme cases, psychosis.

At the other extreme, bipolar depression can feel like "walking underwater with a backpack of stones" or "losing all the colors in the world". It is a tiredness that is not relieved by sleep and a sadness that is not calmed by words of encouragement.

1.4 The Neurochemical Heart of Oscillation

Bipolar disorder is largely a disorder of neurochemical regulation. Alterations in several neurotransmitter systems have been identified:

- **Dopamine:** Excess in mania (hyperactivity, fast thinking) and deficit in depression (apathy, anhedonia).
- **Serotonin:** Fluctuations that influence sleep, appetite, and mood stability.
- **Noradrenaline:** Variations that modulate energy, attention and motivation.
- **Glutamate and GABA:** Imbalances in neuronal excitation and inhibition.

Added to this are alterations in the circadian rhythm, the brain's "internal clock" that regulates when to sleep, eat and be active. That's why sudden changes in sleep schedule can trigger episodes.

1.5 A Common, but Often Invisible Condition

- **Prevalence:** between 1 and 3% of the world's population.
- **Age of onset:** most cases appear between 15 and 25 years old.
- **Diagnostic delay:** it can take up to 7-10 years from the first symptoms to receive the correct diagnosis due to confusions with unipolar depression, attention deficit hyperactivity disorder (ADHD) or personality disorders.
- **Risk of suicide:** Up to 20% of people with bipolar disorder die by suicide if they do not receive proper treatment.

Delayed diagnosis not only delayshelp, but worsens the prognosis: each untreated episode can increase the brain's vulnerability to new episodes.

1.6 Bipolar Disorder in History and Culture

It is no coincidence that we find signs of bipolarity in the lives of figures such as Vincent van Gogh, Virginia Woolf, Ernest Hemingway, Carrie Fisher or Kanye West. In them, bipolarity appears as a double-edged edge: a source of creativity and sensitivity, but also of extreme suffering.

In literature, characters with extreme oscillations have been portrayed as both visionary geniuses and tormented souls. Art, cinema and music have contributed to making visible, but also to distorting the image of this condition.

1.7 The Impact on Everyday Life

Bipolar disorder can affect:

- Personal relationships: breakups, family conflicts, loss of trust.
- Work and studies: low productivity in depression, impulsivity in mania.

- Physical health: sleep disturbances, disordered eating, substance abuse.
- Self-esteem: alternation between feeling invincible and feeling useless.

Without treatment, the life of a person with bipolar disorder can become a succession of reconstructions and losses. With proper treatment it can be a full life, with real control of symptoms.

1.8 The Central Message

Bipolar disorder does not completely define the person who suffers from it. It is a part of their history, but not their entire identity. With correct diagnosis, comprehensive treatment, and consistent support, most people can achieve long periods of stability.

To understand bipolarity is to understand that it is not a matter of turning off the light of mania or ignoring the shadow of depression, but of learning to live between the two, finding firm ground from which to build (Figure 1).

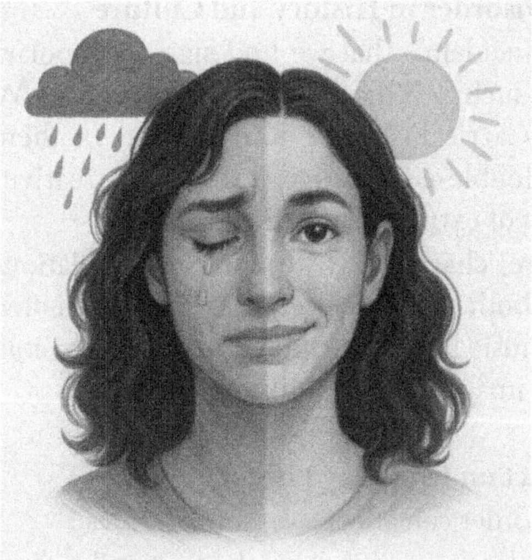

Figure 1. The challenge of living with two poles pulling in opposite directions.

CHAPTER 2
History of Bipolar Disorder: from Greek Melancholy to Modern Stabilization

How we go from humors to mood stabilizers.

2.1 Greece and Rome: Melancholy and Mania as Poles of the Same Phenomenon

- Hippocrates (fifth century B.C.): described melancholia as a state linked to the excess of "black bile" and mania as its hot opposite; he already sensed that both poles were connected.
- Aretaeus of Cappadocia (1st–2nd century A.D.): he made a conceptual leap by arguing that melancholy and mania are part of the same disease with alternating phases.
- Galen (2nd-3rd century A.D.) He consolidated the humoral theory and recommended sleep hygiene, diet and moderation, anticipating, without knowing it, modern pillars.

Keys: early unitary vision, emphasis on rhythms and habits and first "lifestyle" therapies.

2.2 The Middle Ages and the Islamic World: between Demonology and Compassionate Hospitals

- In medieval Europe, the spiritual/demonological reading of madness dominated; custody houses coexisted with coercive practices.
- In the Islamic world, bimaristans (hospitals) offered medical care, music, and baths; Avicenna described states of exaltation and dejection with rational approaches.

Keys: two simultaneous views —moralizing versus medical— with clear ethical implications.

2.3 Renaissance and Enlightenment: from the "Evil of the Soul" to Moral Treatment

- Paracelsus and Burton (Anatomy of Melancholy, 1621) connected body, mind and environment.
- Pinel and Tuke (late eighteenth century) promoted the moral treatment: humanity, routine, work, sleep. They were precursors of psychoeducation.
- Esquirol refined clinical descriptions such as mania and lipemania

Keys: Patient dignity, therapeutic environment and the beginning of the modern clinic.

2.4 Nineteenth Century: Modern Diagnosis is Born

- Falret (1854) describes the *folie circulaire* (cycles of excitement and depression).
- Baillarger (1854) proposes the *folie à double forme* (alternation in the same episode).
- Kraepelin (1899) integrates both into "manic-depressive madness", separating it from dementia praecox (schizophrenia). The unitary conception of bipolar disorder is born.

Keys: bipolarity is consolidated as an entity with a cyclical course and a better prognosis than schizophrenia.

2.5 First Third of the Twentieth Century: Institutionalization and Shock Therapies

- Rise of insane asylums and, sadly, eugenic policies in some countries.
- ECT (Cerletti & Bini, 1938) emerges and, over time, becomes an effective and safe tool (when used with current criteria).
- Episodes of psychosurgery (lobotomy) leave an ethical and clinical wound.

Keys: advances and serious deviations; lessons in bioethics forever.

2.6 The Lithium Revolution

- John Cade (1949) publishes the stabilizing effect of lithium.
- Mogens Schou (1950–1960) demonstrates relapse prevention and reduces suicide risk.
- Once the initial resistance (fear of toxicity) is overcome, lithium becomes a cornerstone with plasma monitoring and renal/thyroid protection.

Keys: first truly prophylactic therapy; the era of stabilization begins.

2.7 Antidepressants and the Recognition of Bipolar II

- With imipramine and MAOI, manic turns appear in vulnerable people; the notion of induced "switch" is born.
- Dunner & Fieve profiled bipolar II disorder in the 1970s: hypomania + major depression (no full-blown mania).
- Interest in cyclothymia and subthreshold spectra is growing.

Keys: the bipolar spectrum expands; caution with antidepressants.

2.8 Atypical Anticonvulsants and Antipsychotics

- Valproate and carbamazepine: useful in mania (and rapid/mixed cycling in some cases).
- Lamotrigine: focus on bipolar depression and maintenance.
- Atypical (olanzapine, quetiapine, risperidone, aripiprazole, lurasidone, cariprazine): efficacy in mania and various options in bipolar depression (e.g., quetiapine, lurasidone, cariprazine).
- Advances in modern ECT, TMS, and more recently, ketamine/esketamine for resistant depression (with strict protocols).

Keys: personalized combinations and monitoring of metabolics, QT, prolactin, weight and extrapyramidal symptoms.

2.9 From DSM-I to DSM-5: Specifying the Language

- DSM-III clearly separates mood disorders and schizophrenia; bipolar I and II are formalized.
- DSM-5 adds specifiers: mixed characteristics, rapid cycling, seasonality, anxiety; reinforces the importance of the longitudinal course.

Keys: better phenotyping = better prognosis and treatment.

2.10 From Categorical to Dimensional Model: the "Bipolar Spectrum"

- Current debate: rigid categories or dimensional continuum (bipolar I cyclothymic ↔ temperament)?
- Opposite risks: overdiagnosis (labeling normal impulses) versus underdiagnosis ("refractory" depressions that were bipolar).
- Importance of circadian rhythms, family burden, previous turns, and response to stabilizers to refine the diagnosis.

Keys: think about trajectories and biographies of mood, not just clinical photos.

2.11 Human Rights, Destigmatization and Community

- Deinstitutionalization (second half of the twentieth century) → rise of community mental health.
- User and family movements: own voice, rights and participation in decisions.
- In Latin America (including Cuba and Mexico): gradual reforms, community networks and a great role for familismo in everyday support.

Keys: treatment is not just a drug; it is a network, dignity and a life project.

2.12 Timeline: Essential Milestones

- s. I–II: Aretaeus proposes mania-melancholy unity.
- 1790–1830: Pinel/Tuke (moral treatment); Esquirol defines paintings.

- 1854: Falret and Baillarger describe cyclical/alternating courses.
- 1899: Kraepelin coins "manic-depressive".
- 1938: Electroconvulsive therapy (Cerletti/Bini).
- 1949–60: Lithium (Cade; Schou) → relapse prevention.
- 1970s: bipolar II (Dunner & Fieve).
- 1990s–2000s: valproate, lamotrigine, atypical; modern guides.
- 2010s–present: refined TMS; ketamine/esketamine; DSM-5 specifiers; personalized medicine.

2.13 Clinical Pearls and Historical Errors that we must not Repeat

Pearls

- Consider bipolar disorder in early-onset depression, antidepressant turns, insomnia with increased energy, family history, and mixed symptoms.
- Sleep is a major therapeutic intervention.
- Lithium remains the gold standard for relapse and suicide prevention (with monitoring).

Mistakes to avoid

- Treat "depression" without exploring a history of hypomania.
- Use antidepressants in monotherapy in probable bipolarity.
- Ignoring circadian factors and family psychoeducation.

The story of bipolar disorder is the story of an ethical and scientific shift: from guilt and confinement to neurobiological understanding, effective treatment, and recovery. Knowing this path inoculates us against stigma and guides us in daily clinical practice (Figure 2).

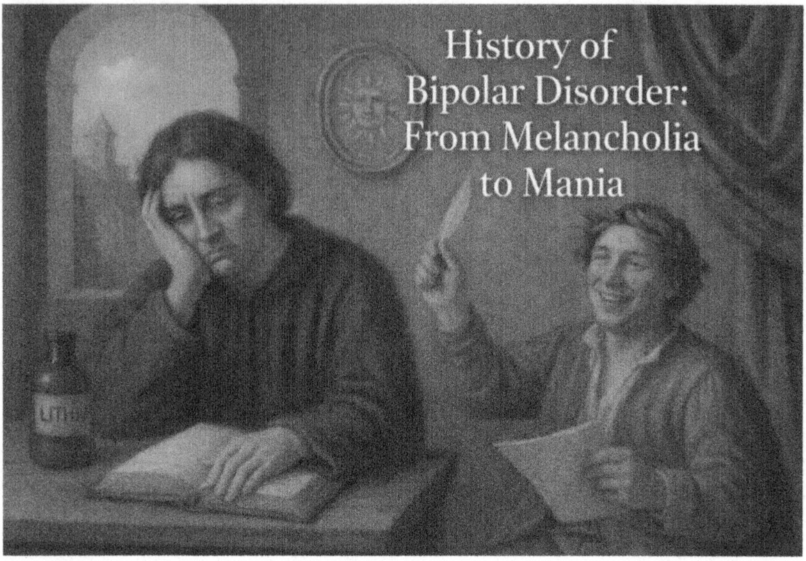

Figure 2. The history of bipolar disorder is the history of an ethical and scientific shift.

CHAPTER 3
Historical and Artistic Characters with Bipolarity: between Genius and Chaos

The creative spark that illuminates and consumes.

3.1 Introduction

The history of humanity is marked by people whose minds seemed to live in two worlds: one of creative euphoria and the other of unfathomable shadows. Bipolar disorder, far from being an "exclusive curse" of the present, has been present in figures who changed the course of art, literature, music and thought. His legacy reminds us that the same energy that can fuel genius can also tear apart personal stability.

This chapter does not seek to idealize suffering or romanticize illness. The aim is to understand how bipolarity influenced the creative process, human relationships and intimate lives of these characters and what lessons we can learn from their stories.

3.2 Vincent van Gogh. The Painter of the Turbulent Soul

In a decade Van Gogh painted more than 2000 works, many in periods of intense creative activity that coincide with what we would today describe as hypomanic or manic phases. His letters to his brother Theo reveal drastic mood swings, prolonged insomnia, and a sense of urgency to create. However, his depressive episodes were devastating, culminating in his suicide at age 37. The intensity of his palette and the movement of his brushstrokes seem to translate the emotional oscillation that he lived internally.

3.3 Virginia Woolf. The Voice that Listened to the Tides of the Mind

The British modernist writer transformed literature with her stream of consciousness style. Woolf alternated periods of inexhaustible literary production with phases of withdrawal, uncontrollable crying and suicidal thoughts.

In her diaries, bipolarity is reflected in entries where she goes from feeling "full of life and vision" to "overwhelmed by a nameless blackness". His death by suicide occurred on March 28, 1941. He left letters in which he asked for forgiveness and described the feeling that "this disease does not let me fight anymore".

3.4 Sylvia Plath. Poetry as a Scalpel of the Soul

Plath turned her pain into sharp, honest verses. His work, especially *Ariel*, reveals oscillations between intense creative energy and paralyzing depressive episodes.

The combination of emotional vulnerability, social pressures, and traumatic personal experiences fueled instability. Plath died at the age of 30 and left an indelible mark on confessional poetry and public awareness of women's mental health.

3.5 Kanye West. Hypermodernity and Real-Time Mania

In the age of social networks, Kanye West has made bipolarity visible like few contemporary artists. He has described his disorder as a "superpower" and, at the same time, has acknowledged the difficulties involved.

His interviews and public episodes reflect impulsiveness, grandiosity, and abrupt mood swings, followed by periods of introspection and media withdrawal.

Her case illustrates how constant exposure and the absence of recovery spaces can exacerbate instability.

3.6 Carrie Fisher. Humor as a Lifesaver

The actress and writer, famous for her role as Princess Leia, spoke openly about her bipolarity and substance addiction. With an ironic and demystifying approach, Fisher fought stigma and gave motivational talks about living with and working with the disease.

His legacy is not only artistic, but educational: he taught that bipolarity does not define a person, and that it is possible to combine medical treatment, self-acceptance and creativity.

3.7 Conclusions

These cases show that bipolar disorder does not manifest itself identically in each person. Creativity is not a direct consequence of the disease, but its cycles can influence the way in which the artistic work is perceived and produced.

Behind the admiration for genius, it is crucial to recognize the need for treatment, social support, and self-care strategies so that talent is not consumed in the fire of instability (Figure 3).

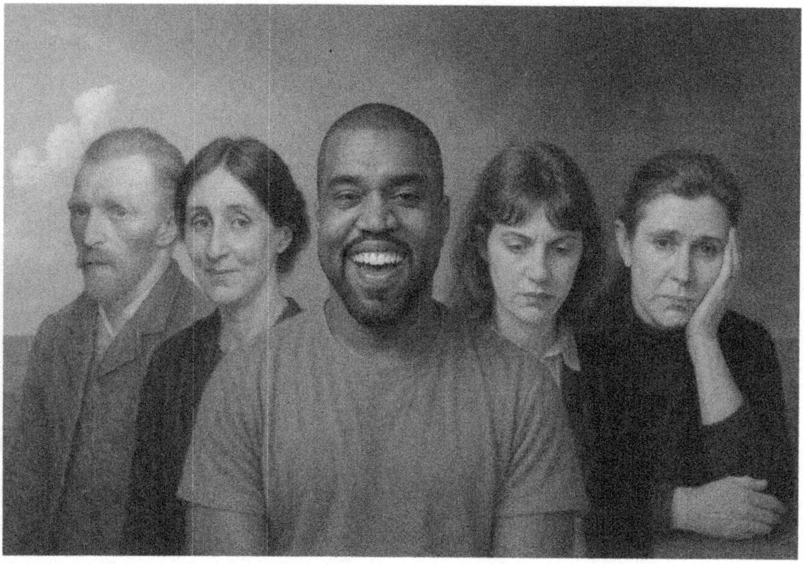

Figure 3. When the creative light and the inner shadow coexist in the same mind. Between genius and chaos: historical minds that lived with bipolarity.

CHAPTER 4
Depictions in Film, Literature and Music

How has bipolar disorder been portrayed and understood through art and media?

4.1 The Power of Art to Make Bipolarity Visible

Art has been one of the most powerful vehicles to bring the experience of bipolar disorder to the general public. Through film, literature and music, stories have been told that explore the complexity of living with this condition, showing its emotional extremes and its impacts on creativity, relationships and mental health.

These representations, although sometimes stereotyped, open doors to empathy, reflection and destigmatization. However, they can also reinforce myths if they are not done with rigor and scientific respect.

4.2 Bipolarity in Cinema: Realism, Drama and Stigma

Cinema has addressed bipolarity in various genres, from biographical drama to black comedy. Some films have achieved deep and clinically accurate portraits, while others have exaggerated or distorted aspects to generate emotional impact.

Emblematic films:

- *Mr. Jones* (1993): Based on the true story of a journalist with bipolar disorder, this film offers a human and complex look at mania and depression, including the therapeutic process.
- *Silver Linings Playbook* (2012): Winner of an Oscar, it portrays the life of a man with bipolarity who seeks to rebuild his life and relationships, combining humor and realism.
- *The Hours* (2002): Inspired by the life of Virginia Woolf, it explores the emotional suffering and creativity linked to mental illness.

- *Infinitely Polar Bear* (2014): Dramatic comedy showing the impact of bipolar disorder on family life and parenthood.

4.2.1 Science and Myth in Cinema

Films have the power to educate, but also the responsibility not to fall into stigmas. Bipolarity is not synonymous with violence or extreme madness; it is a medical condition that can be managed with treatment. Showing the full spectrum, including stable phases and remissions, helps correct misperceptions.

4.3 Literature: the Inner Voice of Bipolar Disorder

Literature has been a refuge and a mirror for those who live with bipolarity. Writers such as Virginia Woolf, Sylvia Plath and Kay Redfield Jamison have masterfully captured the inner tumult and complex beauty of the disorder.

- Virginia Woolf in her diaries and novels expressed the fluidity and emotional chaos that characterize bipolarity, with a sensitivity that has inspired generations.
- Sylvia Plath, through her poetry and the novel *The Bell Jar*, spoke openly about bipolar depression and suicide, mixing pain and creation.
- Kay Redfield Jamison, clinical psychologist and patient, has published scientific and autobiographical works that combine rigor and emotion, being an authoritative voice to understand the disease from the inside and outside.

Literature allows unique access to subjectivity, where sensations, thoughts, and emotions that clinical tools do not always capture can be explored.

4.4 Music: Rhythm, Emotion and Bipolarity

Music has been both a refuge and an expression of bipolar disorder for many artists. From classics to contemporaries, numerous musicians have spoken publicly about their bipolarity and have reflected it in their lyrics, rhythms and presentations.

- Kurt Cobain (Nirvana) and Björk have been linked to experiences of bipolarity and have channeled their sensibility into iconic works.
- Michael Jackson and Mariah Carey spoke openly about their diagnoses, which helped normalize the topic in show business.
- Rapper Kanye West, a contemporary example of how bipolarity can influence creativity and public life, has faced stigma with honesty and controversy.

Music can reflect the alternation between mania and depression, the fast-paced pace of thought, or deep sadness, helping others feel like they're not alone.

4.5 Impact on Social Perception and Current Challenges

Artistic and media representations influence the social perception of bipolar disorder, for better or worse. Visibility has increased awareness, but clichés and exaggerations persist.

Among the challenges is to achieve an image that combines:

- Clinical accuracy: Recognizing the complexity and diversity of the bipolar spectrum.
- Humanization: showing people as full subjects and not as "cases" or "patients".
- Hope and recovery: Emphasize that with treatment and support, stability is possible.

4.6 What to Learn from these Representations?

- Art can be a bridge to empathy and education.
- Bipolarity is not just a drama or a comedy but a multifaceted condition that requires a multidimensional approach.
- Real stories, authentic voices and scientific rigor must be allies to demystify and destigmatize.

4.7 Conclusion

Film, literature and music offer privileged windows to understand bipolar disorder beyond manuals. They invite us to listen to human complexity, to recognize the suffering and beauty that coexist in bipolarity, and to build bridges that allow a full and dignified life for those who live it.

CHAPTER 5
Types of Bipolar Disorder: Bipolar I, II, Cyclothymia and Intermediate Spectra

Between euphoria and the abyss: cartography of extreme moods.

5.1 The Diversity of the Same Fire

No two bipolars are the same. There are those who burn and burn away; others only spark and return to balance; Some seem to live a normal life until, suddenly, an invisible wave changes its course.

Bipolarity, more than a single disease, is a territory with mountains, hills and emotional valleys. Understanding their clinical types is equivalent to studying a map: not to label, but to guide the traveler and prevent abysses.

Every medical classification has a practical purpose: knowing the intensity, frequency and duration of the episodes allows the treatment to be personalized.

Thus, the psychiatrist ceases to be a firefighter who puts out fires to become a meteorologist of the soul, capable of anticipating storms and teaching the patient to navigate.

5.2 Bipolar Disorder Type I. The Summit of Lightning

Bipolar Iis the most visible form, the one that often breaks into the emergency room or family news. Its hallmark is the manic episode: an expansion of energy so powerful that it can raise productivity and creativity to extraordinary levels... or overflow all containment.

Clinical manifestations

- Expansive euphoria or intense irritability.
- Hyperactivity: Almost total insomnia without fatigue.
- Flight of ideas: quick thoughts, accelerated speech.

- Great self-esteem: "I am chosen", "everything makes sense".
- Impulsivity: spending, promiscuity, alcohol abuse, decisions without calculation.
- Psychotic symptoms in severe cases: delusions of power, divine or paranoid voices.

In the manic phase, critical judgment disappears; the individual feels that anything is possible, and his environment suffers the consequences.

Clinical case 1: "The project of the century"

María, 32 years old, art teacher.

One morning he began to paint murals throughout the school "to awaken the aesthetic conscience of the country". He had not slept for five nights and spoke at a hypnotic speed. When he arrived at the emergency room he said: "God dictated a national educational plan to me". After managing to stabilize it with lithium, his talent was not extinguished; he simply learned to use fire with gloves.

Neurochemical explanation

During mania there is an excess of dopamine and glutamate in the limbic system, while GABA (the natural brake) decreases. The brain accelerates like an engine without a clutch: it turns brilliantly, but also with the risk of explosion.

Treatment and Prognosis

Management focuses on mood stabilizers (lithium, valproate) and atypical antipsychotics. The goal is to prevent relapse and protect sleep, since a single sleepless night can rekindle the storm.

5.3 Bipolar Disorder Type II. The Silent Fire

Bipolar II is more discreet.

Their hypomanias can pass as "productive times" or "good times", but they hide a risk: the higher you climb uncontrollably, the deeper the descent.

Features

- Episodes of hypomania of at least 4 days.
- High energy, increased sociability, intense creativity.
- No psychotic symptoms or hospitalization.
- Prolonged and severe depressions afterwards.

Clinical case 2: "The Luminous Programmer"

Luis, a software engineer, could work 20 hours straight "without feeling tired". He published three projects in one week, convinced that he had "finally understood the code of the universe". Two weeks later, he couldn't get up, or answer emails, or look in the mirror. The diagnosis of bipolar II changed his life: he stopped hating his cycles and began to organize his energy.

5.4 The Emotional Paradox

The bipolar II patient usually feels guilty for his sadness because he remembers with nostalgia the clarity of his hypomania. That's why many try to "self-induce" energy with caffeine, sleepless nights or multiple projects... aggravating the imbalance.

Clinical Management

Lamotrigine, quetiapine or lurasidone are useful drugs to stabilize depression without causing mania. Psychological accompaniment is crucial: teaching the patient not to romanticize their hypomania.

5.5 Cyclothymia. The Subtle Swing

Cyclothymia is a small pendulum that never stops. The emotions are not extreme, but there is no rest: every week an oscillation. It does not cause hospitalization, but it does cause existential fatigue.

Clinical case 3: "The invisible roller coaster"

Andrea, 27, a graphic designer, alternated days of enthusiasm with others of irritability and apathy. Her partners called her "intense"; her bosses said she "shines, sometimes she disappears". In reality, he was living through cyclothymia: small chemical storms that never became hurricanes, but got wet every day.

Neurophysiology

Cyclothymia involves dopaminergic and serotonergic micro-fluctuations. The limbic system overreacts to everyday stimuli; The biological clock is easily mismatched.

Treatment

More than suppressing emotions, it seeks to synchronize rhythms:

- Regular sleep.
- Daily exercise.
- Social rhythm-focused psychotherapy (IPSRT).
- Small doses of stabilizers.

"Cyclothymia is like living on a coast where every day there is high or low tide, but never total calm".

5.6 Mixed Forms and Fast Cycles. When the Soul Runs and Cries at the Same Time

Mixed episodes

The patient laughs and cries at the same time. He has the energy to move, but his thinking is dark; he feels guilt and at the same time suicidal impulses. The danger is maximum: the energy of mania coupled with the pain of depression.

Fast cycles

They are diagnosed when there are four or more episodes in a year. They can be seen in women, in hypothyroidism, or by inappropriate use of antidepressants. The brain seems to lose its internal compass: each hormonal change, each night badly slept, triggers a new cycle.

Management

- Avoid antidepressants without a stabilizer.
- Regulate sleep and hormones.
- Circadian rhythm therapy and mood diary.

5.7 Art, Literature and the Types of Bipolarity

Culture has unknowingly reflected these subtypes.

- Bipolar I: Van Gogh, in his letters to Theo, describes fiery manias followed by nights of emptiness.
- Bipolar II: Virginia Woolf alternated periods of creative lucidity with immense depressions: "The wave rises, the wave falls, and between the two I try to write".
- Cyclothymia: Truman Capote and his mild but constant emotional instability; his friends said he had "champagne days and quiet days".

Art becomes a mirror: it allows us to understand that bipolarity is not only a disorder, but an extreme form of humanity (Table 1).

Table 1. Clinical Comparison of Major Subtypes of Bipolar Disorder

Type	Bipolar I	Bipolar II	Cyclothymia	Mixed/ Fast
Episode Length	≥ 7 days mania	≥ 4 days hypomania + depression	≥ 2 years slight fluctuations	Variable
Intensity	High	Media	Low	Very high
Functional Risk	Serious	Moderate	Mild	Serious
Psychotic Symptoms	Possible	No	No	Possible
Predominance	Euphoria/ irritability	Depression	Variable	Combined
Frequent Relapses	Yes	Yes	Frequent	Very common
Base Treatment	Lithium + antipsychotic	Lamotrigina, quetiapina	Therapy + low stabilizer	Tight combination

5.8 The Family and Social Perspective

Many families take years to recognize bipolarity because each type generates a different narrative:

- In bipolar I, the environment is frightened.
- In bipolar II, it is confused with perfectionism or depression.
- In cyclothymia, it is labeled as "changing character".

Family psychoeducation teaches that it is not laziness or evil, but emotional biology. When the inner circle understands this, the prognosis improves dramatically.

Practical Advice for Patients:

- Keep a daily mood log (1-10).
- Don't chase euphoria. Stability may seem boring, but it is freedom.
- Protects sleep: it is your natural stabilizer.
- Avoid alcohol, stimulants and sleepless nights.
- Learn to recognize early signs: speech acceleration, less need for sleep, irritability, multiple plans.
- Let your family or therapist know before the episode escalates.
- Accept medication as part of balance, not punishment.

5.9 The Map of Bipolarity

Knowing the type of bipolarity that one suffers from is like learning to read one's own inner climate. Bipolar I faces thunderstorms; bipolar II, persistent rains; cyclothymia, a changing sky every day.

But in all cases, knowledge and structure can turn prognosis into hope. The diagnosis is not a condemnation: it is the map that allows you to return home whenever your mood goes astray (Figure 4).

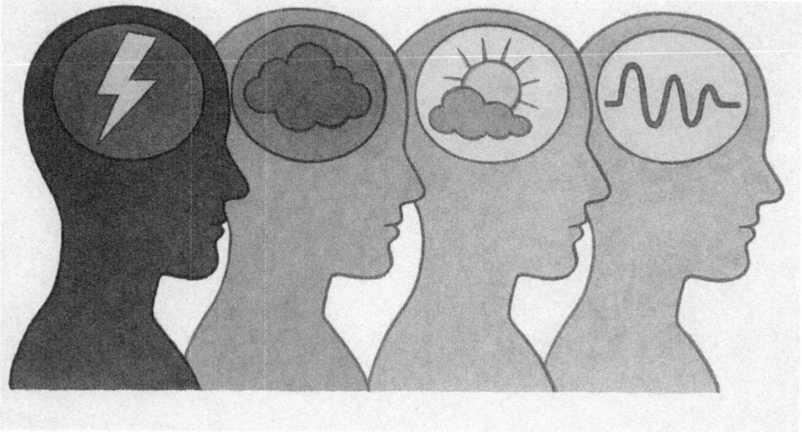

Figure 4. Conceptual representation of the bipolar spectrum: from the electrical intensity of mania to the darkness of depression, and finally to the balanced rhythm of emotional stability. The image symbolizes how each phase is part of a single human continuum, rather than separate identities.

CHAPTER 6
Common Myths and Common Diagnostic Errors

Dismantling prejudices: between social stigma and clinical confusion.

6.1 When the Myth Disguises itself as Truth

Bipolar disorder is one of the most misunderstood conditions in modern psychiatry. Despite advances in neuroscience, society —and sometimes even health professionals— continue to be trapped in simplistic or misconceptions that distort their understanding.

The word "bipolar" has been trivialized to the point of becoming an everyday adjective. It is used to describe someone who is changing, temperamental or unstable: "today he is happy, tomorrow sad, he is bipolar".

This trivialization has contributed to millions of real patients being made invisible or stigmatized, and medical diagnosis being misused. Demolishing myths is an essential step to humanize treatment and restore the dignity of those who live with bipolarity.

6.2 Myth 1: "We're all a Little Bipolar"

No, not all of us are. We all experience mood swings, but in bipolar those changes are extreme, pathological, and disproportionate. They involve a profound alteration of neurotransmitters, sleep, vital energy and judgment.

The bipolar brain doesn't change moods on a whim, but because its internal regulation of pleasure, motivation, and stress works differently. To say that "we are all bipolar" is like saying that "we are all diabetic because we sometimes eat sugar".

The result of this myth is serious: it minimizes the patient's real suffering and delays the search for professional help.

6.3 Myth 2: "Bipolar People are Dangerous"

The danger is not in the person, but in the untreated crisis. During a manic or psychotic episode there may be impulsivity, disinhibition or irritability, but in the vast majority of cases the patient is not violent, but vulnerable, disorganized and scared.

In reality, people with bipolar disorder are at greater risk of harming themselves than others. The stigma of the "dangerous bipolar" fuels social fear and hinders work, academic and family integration.

When treated, followed, and understood, bipolar patients are often responsible, empathetic, and highly creative.

6.4 Myth 3: "Drugs Turn off Personality"

One of the most frequent fears. The patient fears losing his energy, his spark, his identity. But what drugs really do is reduce the extremes, not erase the essence.

Lithium or lamotrigine do not eliminate creativity; they eliminate the impulsivity that destroys the work. Chemical balance does not silence the soul, it harmonizes it.

When the treatment is well adjusted, the person does not feel "annulled", but more aware, more in control of themselves. The purpose of psychiatry is not to turn off the light, but to prevent the filament from burning.

6.5 Myth 4: "Bipolar Disorder is Cured with Willpower"

The will is valuable, but insufficient. Bipolar disorder is a chronic medical illness, with genetic, neurochemical and environmental bases. Denying it in the name of self-control is as absurd as asking an asthmatic to breathe without an inhaler or a diabetic to regulate their glucose with optimism.

Willpower helps to follow treatment, maintain habits and ask for help; but it is not a substitute for treatment.

6.6 Myth 5: "Bipolar is just a Form of Depression"

This mistake is common, even among professionals. Many people with bipolar disorder spend years diagnosed with unipolar depression. The problem arises when they receive antidepressants without a mood stabilizer: dopamine rises uncontrollably and can trigger mania or a rapid cycle.

It is estimated that between 30 and 50% of patients initially treated as depressive actually belong to the bipolar spectrum. The fundamental difference lies in the cyclical pattern and longitudinal history of the patient.

The psychiatrist should always ask:

"Have there been times when you felt too energetic, slept too little, and saw everything too clearly?"

The answer to that question can change an entire diagnosis.

6.7 Common Clinical Error: Confusing Bipolar with ADHD or Borderline

Bipolar versus ADHD

Both share impulsivity, distractibility, and variable energy, but ADHD is constant, while bipolar is episodic. Bipolar can have weeks of total calm between phases; ADHD cannot.

Bipolar versus borderline personality disorder

In the borderline, emotional oscillations are reactive to bonds, last for hours or days, and arise from affective wounds. In bipolarity, the changes are endogenous, of neurochemical origin, and last for weeks or months.

Distinguishing the two conditions is essential because the treatments are completely different.

6.8 Common Clinical Error: Underestimating the Role of Sleep and Hormones

Many bipolar episodes begin with a sleep disturbance: sleeping less, dreaming more vividly, waking up earlier. Sleep is the most faithful thermometer of the bipolar brain.

Likewise, hormonal changes (pregnancy, postpartum, thyroid, menopause) can alter emotional stability. That is why the follow-up must be interdisciplinary: psychiatry, endocrinology, family medicine.

6.9 The Impact of Stigma

Beyond biology, the social burden is enormous. Being called "bipolar" is used as an insult or mockery. The patient learns to hide their symptoms and to pretend normality, developing guilt and shame.

Stigma not only hurts: it kills, because it takes away from treatment. Speaking respectfully, teaching, and showing examples of stable living is an act of prevention.

6.10 Re-educating the Gaze

Bipolarity is not a weakness or a moral disorder. It is a human condition that demands understanding, science, and compassion. Each myth that is dismantled opens space for a real story of recovery. Scientific knowledge heals the mind; empathy heals the soul.

6.11 Final Recommendations for Professionals

- Listen to the full story, not just the current episode.
- Investigate family history and previous energy changes.
- Do not lightly label it with "personality disorder".
- Explain the diagnosis in human, not technical, language.
- Incorporate the family environment from the beginning.

6.12 Conclusion

Understanding bipolarity does not mean justifying its crises, but accompanying its oscillating nature with respect and medical precision. Stigma and diagnostic errors don't just hurt; distort the patient's truth.

Modern psychiatry must recover its most human gaze: the one that sees in each cycle not a chemical scandal, but an attempt by the brain to rediscover its inner rhythm. Knowledge does not label: it illuminates (Figure 5).

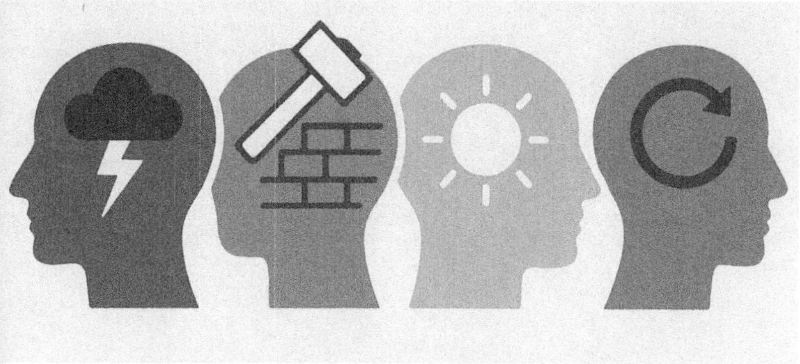

Figure 5. Conceptual representation of the dismantling of myths and diagnostic confusion around bipolar disorder. The image transitions from darkness to clarity, symbolizing the journey from stigma and misinterpretation to understanding, science, and compassion.

PART II.
Neurobiological and Neurochemical bases

CHAPTER 7
The Bipolar Brain: Regions Involved in Mania and Depression

The neurochemical dance between euphoria and inner silence.

7.1 The Internal Mood Scenario

If we could observe the bipolar brain in the middle of an episode, we would see a fascinating and stormy spectacle: areas that light up like lightning and others that go out like deserts.

Each mood change corresponds to a change in the activity of specific neural networks. Bipolar disorder is not just an emotional disturbance, but a cerebral dysrhythmia: the circuits that regulate energy, pleasure, judgment, and motivation lose synchrony.

Understanding which areas of the brain are involved in mania and depression allows us to get closer to the mystery of why the same mind can shine brightly and then fall into darkness.

7.2 The Emotional Brain: The Symphony of the Limbic System

The limbic system is the emotional heart of the brain. It includes structures such as the amygdala, hippocampus, anterior cingulate, and hypothalamus.

In bipolarity, these regions function like an orchestra without a conductor: each instrument plays with a different rhythm.

- Amygdala: regulates fear, anger, and emotional intensity. In mania, his activity increases; in depression, it is extinguished.
- Hippocampus: stores memories and experiences. In depressive phases it can reduce its volume due to excess cortisol, while in mania it is hyperactive with accelerated associations.

- Anterior cincture: bridge between emotion and reason. When dysregulation occurs, impulsivity, guilt, or lack of control appear.
- Hypothalamus: Regulates sleep, appetite, and circadian rhythm; its imbalance explains drastic changes in energy and sleep.

Together, these structures transform emotional experience into biology. The limbic system is the voice of the soul translated into electrical impulses.

7.3 The Prefrontal Cortex: The Regulator of Judgment

Under normal conditions, the dorsolateral prefrontal cortex functions as a "moral brake" that modulates impulses. During mania, this brake is weakened: the patient thinks quickly, acts without measuring consequences, feels omnipotent. Neuroimaging shows prefrontal hypoactivity and limbic hyperactivity, an explosive combination.

In depression, the opposite happens: the prefrontal cortex becomes overloaded with negative thoughts, hyperanalyzes every mistake and loses the ability to hope. The balance between prefrontal (reason) and limbic (emotion) is the key to mental well-being.

7.4 The Basal Ganglia and the Reward Circuit

The basal ganglia —especially the nucleus accumbens and striatum— are responsible for pleasure, motivation, and the urge to act. In mania, they release excess dopamine, which generates a feeling of invincibility and euphoria.

The world seems bright, the colors intense, the ideas possible. In depression, the opposite phenomenon occurs: dopaminergic deficit. Everything feels flat, slow, without reward.

This dopaminergic alternation explains why many patients describe their state as "on or off", with no nuances in between.

7.5 The HPA Axis and Chronic Stress

The hypothalamic-pituitary-adrenal (HPA) axis is the system that coordinates the stress response. In bipolarity, this shaft behaves like a damaged spring: it overreacts or does not react at all.

- In mania: increased cortisol and adrenaline → hyperalertness, insomnia, energy expenditure.
- In depression: exhaustion of the axis → fatigue, anhedonia, mental slowness.

Over time, oscillations of the HPA axis alter neuroplasticity and the immune system, which explains why bipolar patients have greater systemic inflammation and physical vulnerability.

7.6 Neural Networks Involved

Modern neuroscience no longer speaks only of structures, but of functional networks:

- Default mode network (DMN): overactive in depression → excessive introspection, rumination, and guilt.
- Executive network: hypoactive in mania → loss of control and planning.
- Salience network: overactivated in both phases → extreme sensitivity to stimuli.

The bipolar brain alternates between hyperconnection and disconnection, as if emotional wires are plugged in and unplugged without warning.

7.7 Neuroimaging: the Visual Signature of Bipolar Disorder

The techniques of fMRI (functional resonance imaging) and PET (positron emission tomography) have shown clear differences:

- In mania: increased blood flow in the amygdala, thalamus, and orbitofrontal cortex; reduced prefrontal control.
- In depression : lower activity in the dorsolateral cortex, lower metabolism of the frontal lobe and hippocampus.

These patterns are so consistent that some researchers are already talking about a brain signature of the bipolar spectrum, an electrical fingerprint that distinguishes internal oscillation from normal neurochemical balance.

7.8 Cerebral Laterality and Bipolar Creativity

The right hemisphere —more intuitive and artistic— is activated with greater intensity during manic phases, while the left hemisphere —more logical and analytical— predominates in depression.

This hemispheric alternation could explain why many people with bipolarity show outstanding creative talent in periods of stability.

Creativity is not born from illness, but from the contact between chaos and order that the patient learns to translate into art, writing or invention. Bipolar genius does not lie in mania, but in the lucidity that follows the storm.

7.9 Brain Plasticity and Therapeutic Hope

The bipolar brain was long believed to be structurally defective. Today we know that it is plastic and adaptable. With treatment, adequate sleep, and chemical stability, hippocampal volume can recover, functional connectivity improved, and inflammation decreased.

The bipolar brain is not broken: it is in constant adjustment. Each episode leaves scars, yes, but also new paths for resilience.

7.10 The Inner Dance

Bipolar disorder is a brain choreography, where emotion, judgment, and memory take turns to dominate the scene. In mania, the fire rises; In depression, water floods. But at the midpoint, when both elements are balanced, consciousness appears.

Understanding the bipolar brain not only allows us to treat it better: it invites us to reconcile ourselves with the biology of emotion, with the idea that each thought has its rhythm, and each mood, its anatomy. The mind is not a battleground between reason and madness: it is the living language of the brain seeking balance between its lights and shadows (Figure 6).

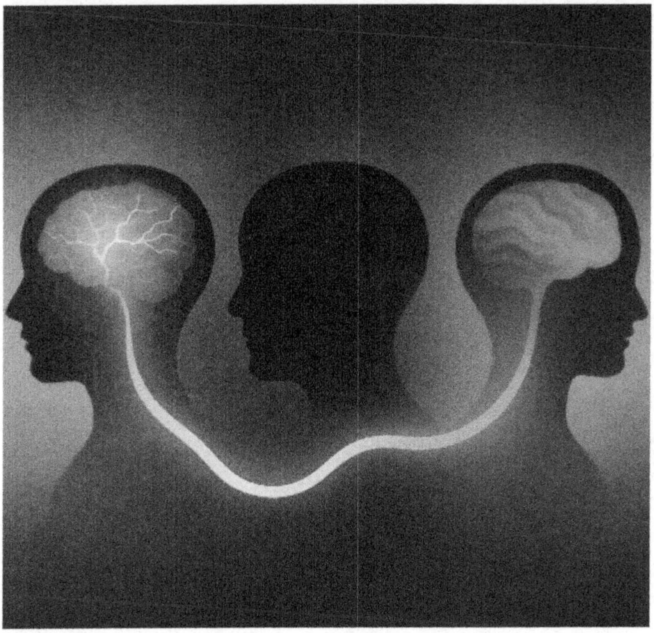

Figure 6. Conceptual representation of the bipolar brain, where one side radiates the electrical energy of mania and the other is immersed in the cold stillness of depression. The central figure symbolizes balance: the restoration of neural rhythm and emotional harmony.

CHAPTER 8
Key Neurotransmitters: Dopamine, Serotonin, Glutamate, GABA, Norepinephrine and more

The invisible messengers of the human soul.

8.1 The Chemistry that Thinks us

The bipolar brain can be understood as a symphony of chemical messengers that, instead of acting in harmony, are out of sync. Each neurotransmitter represents an instrument: dopamine plays the violins of motivation, serotonin sets the pace of well-being, GABA keeps the background calm, and glutamate provides the intensity of the brass.

When one is accelerated or silenced, the emotional melody is distorted.

Understanding these messengers is essential for every psychiatrist: neurochemistry is the most intimate language of the mood.

8.2 Dopamine. The Fuel of Euphoria and Creativity

Dopamine regulates motivation, pleasure, and reward. In mania, its release increases uncontrollably, especially in the nucleus accumbens and the prefrontal cortex. The patient feels brilliant, powerful, with ideas that flow relentlessly.

Clinical example

During his manic phase, Alejandro —a 29 years old musician— composed ten songs in a week. He hardly slept. He spoke fast, convinced that he had discovered a new musical genre. His brain, flooded with dopamine, drove him to create without pause, but also to spend his money on instruments he didn't need.

Dopamine is like the gasoline in a sports engine: it offers power, but if you press the accelerator without brakes, the vehicle goes off the road. In depression, the opposite happens: the dopaminergic system shuts down. The same activities that once produced pleasure now seem hollow. The patient says "nothing excites me anymore", thus reflecting a true motivational blackout.

8.3 Serotonin. The Architect of Emotional Balance

Serotonin modulates mood, sleep, appetite, and impulsivity. In bipolar, it fluctuates like a pendulum. When it decreases, irritability, insomnia and hopelessness appear; When it increases along with dopamine, euphoria and mental acceleration arise.

Clinical case

Laura, 36 years old, had recurrent depressions treated with SSRI antidepressants. After an increase in dosage, he developed insomnia, verbiage, and a sense of omnipotence. His diagnosis of bipolar II had gone unnoticed.

Excess serotonin without dopaminergic stabilization precipitated hypomania. The psychiatrist must remember that serotonin is not "the happiness hormone", but a control module that, when interacting with dopamine, can lead to both calm and agitation.

8.4 Noradrenaline. The Energy of the Alert

Norepinephrine (or norepinephrine) comes from the locus coeruleus and regulates attention, drive, and stress response. During mania, it is over-released, leading to hyperalertness, tachycardia, and cascading thinking. In depression, its deficit causes mental slowness, fatigue and low concentration.

Imagine the noradrenergic system as a biological accelerator: the right amount maintains attention and performance; excess generates anxiety and deficit, apathy. For this reason, many modern stabilizers and antipsychotics seek to balance dopamine and norepinephrine, allowing the patient to regain energy without losing control.

8.5 GABA. The Brain Brake

GABA (gamma-aminobutyric acid) is the main inhibitory neurotransmitter. Its function is to calm excessive neural activity. In mania, GABA levels decrease: the brain loses its natural brake. In depression, it can increase too much, generating a dull emotional tone and cognitive slowness.

Drugs that potentiate GABA —such as certain benzodiazepines or valproate— help to stabilize excitation peaks, although their use should be prudent to avoid dependence or excessive sedation. GABA is the silence that allows the neural orchestra not to become noise.

8.6 Glutamate. The Spark of Arousal

Glutamate is the most abundant excitatory neurotransmitter in the brain.

During mania, its release is triggered; neurons communicate so quickly that thinking speeds up. In depression, its poor regulation reduces synaptic plasticity and contributes to the feeling of "sluggish mind".

The discovery of glutamate-modulating drugs, such as ketamine and esketamine, has revolutionized the treatment of resistant bipolar depression, by offering rapid antidepressant effects through the restoration of synaptic connectivity.

8.7 Other Couriers Involved

Acetylcholine

It is involved in memory, sleep, and mood regulation. Their increase in depression can intensify excessive introspection.

Endorphins and oxytocin

They affect the sensation of pleasure and affective bonding. Many bipolar patients improve markedly when they achieve emotional reconnection and human contact because oxytocin acts as a natural stabilizer.

Cortisol and stress hormones

Its chronic elevation alters hippocampal function and accelerates the cycles of the disorder, linking the biology of stress with mood swing.

8.8 Interactions and Balance

Neurotransmitters do not act in isolation. Dopamine stimulates, GABA slows down. Serotonin modulates, norepinephrine awakens, and glutamate ignites the spark. Its dynamic balance creates the emotional tone.

The therapeutic challenge is to synchronize the chemical orchestra, not to silence its instruments. Every treatment —be it lithium, valproate, antipsychotic, or psychodynamic therapy— seeks to restore that invisible harmony.

8.9 Integrative Example

In a typical manic episode:

- Dopamine and norepinephrine increase → hyperenergy.
- Glutamate is triggered → accelerated thinking.
- GABA and serotonin lower → loss of control and insomnia.

In bipolar depression:

- Dopamine and norepinephrine lower → apathy.
- GABA and serotonin increase → emotional inhibition.
- Glutamate drops or becomes toxic → cognitive slowness.

These patterns allow precise treatments to be designed to dose the balance between arousal and calm.

8.10 Modern Therapeutic Perspective

The future of bipolar treatment points towards personalized neurochemistry. Genetic analysis and pharmacogenomics will allow us to identify which dopaminergic or serotonergic pathways predominate in each patient.

It will no longer be "bipolar depression type I or II", but dominant neurochemical profiles. The DNP-21, as a clinical instrument, seeks just that: to translate symptoms into neurotransmission profiles to guide treatment towards biological precision (Figure 7).

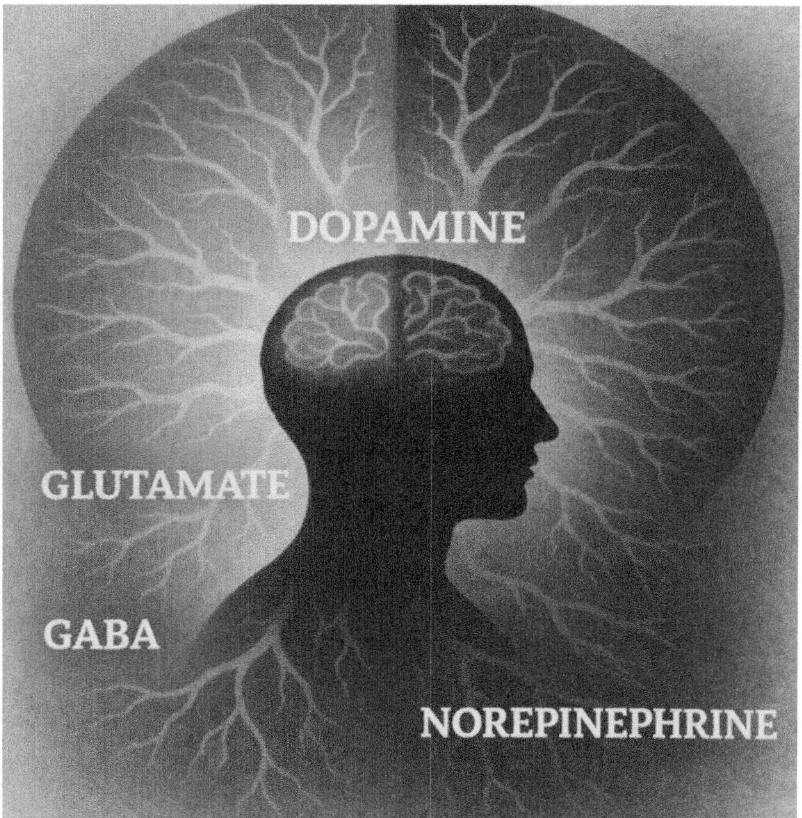

Figure 7. Conceptual representation of the main neurotransmitters involved in bipolar disorder. The warm and cold hemispheres symbolize the dynamic balance between excitation and inhibition: dopamine, glutamate, GABA, and noradrenaline in constant interaction to maintain the emotional rhythm.

8.11 The Messengers of the Soul

Neurotransmitters are the words with which the brain writes emotions. Her invisible dance defines how we love, think, remember and dream. In bipolar disorder, that dance speeds up or stops, but it never dies out.

To understand its movements is to understand humanity itself: the chemistry that thinks us, the biology that feels us, and the soul that seeks balance in the midst of both.

CHAPTER 9
Circadian Rhythm, Sleep-Wake Cycle and Seasonal Dysregulation

When the internal beat loses its compass.

9.1 The Biological Clock of the Soul

The human body has an invisible clock that marks each of its functions: temperature, hormonal secretion, hunger, sleep, energy, attention. That clock —the circadian rhythm— beats in nearly every cell and is directed by a tiny structure in the brain called the suprachiasmatic nucleus, located in the hypothalamus.

In most people, this system syncs with sunlight and daily routines. But in bipolar disorder, that clock is moving forward or backward, leading to profound alterations in mood and cognition.

The bipolar brain is a clock that keeps ticking the right time... in the wrong time zone.

9.2 Circadian Rhythm and Mood

Studies show that bipolar patients have abnormalities in the expression of circadian genes such as CLOCK, BMAL1 and PER3, which regulate the production of melatonin, cortisol and neurotransmitters. When these genes are mismatched, the brain loses the ability to accurately distinguish between day and night, activity and rest, excitement and calm.

That's why many patients describe their mania as "a night that never ends" and their depression as "a dawn that never comes".

9.3 Sleep: The Bipolar Balance Thermometer

Sleep is the sentinel symptom of bipolar disorder. Before a manic episode, it usually subsides; Before a depression, it can be prolonged. A single change in sleep pattern can herald the onset of a crisis.

Clinical case

Samuel, 40 years old, had been stable for two years with maintenance treatment. One week, due to night work, he slept just four hours a day. At first he felt an "incredible energy", but soon he began to speak quickly, to spend money and to feel that "everything had a special meaning".

Insomnia had acted as a chemical detonator: his circadian rhythm lost pace. Sleep is not a biological luxury; It is the mechanism that repairs neurotransmitters and synchronizes the cortex with the limbic system.

9.4 Melatonin and Light: the Guardians of the Internal Clock

Melatonin, a hormone secreted by the pineal gland during darkness, acts as a nighttime signal to the body.

In bipolar patients, their release is usually delayed or reduced, leading to insomnia, nocturnal activation, and difficulty mentally disconnecting.

Exposure to light —natural or artificial— directly influences its production. For this reason, controlled phototherapy and light hygiene have become complementary therapeutic tools.

Clinical strategies:

- Avoid bright screens at least an hour before bedtime.
- Daily sun exposure of 20 to 30 minutes.
- Use of white light lamps in the morning in seasonal depressions.
- Maintain regular schedules, even on weekends.

9.5 Hormonal Rhythms and Seasons of the Year

The human mood has seasons, and in bipolarity those seasons are intensified. Autumn and winter are usually associated with a higher risk of depression, while spring and summer favour hypomanic or manic episodes.

Changes in light, temperature, and length of day modify the secretion of melatonin, cortisol, and serotonin. It's as if the bipolar brain were an exaggerated atmospheric sensor: it senses the brightest sunrise and the darkest sunset than the rest.

The human body was designed for daylight and the silence of night. When the biological clock is reversed, the soul also loses its north.

9.6 Chronotherapy and Sleep-Wake Regulation

Chronotherapy seeks to restore the natural rhythm through non-pharmacological interventions:

- Partial sleep deprivation: used in resistant bipolar depressions (under medical supervision).
- Morning phototherapy: simulates sunrise and regulates melatonin secretion.
- Schedule control: always getting up and going to bed at the same time.
- Avoid prolonged naps: they keep the circadian axis active and prevent relapses (Figure 8).

In parallel, mood stabilizers (such as lithium) also act on circadian genes, which explains why their regular use improves both sleep and emotional stability.

9.7 Interaction between Sleep, Neurotransmitters and Episodes

During deep sleep, dopamine and serotonin levels are rebalanced, while GABA modulates neuronal excitation.

When sleep is interrupted, dopamine increases and serotonin falls: the brain interprets this desynchronization as a manic stimulus.

Mania is, in many ways, a state of perpetual wakefulness; depression, a state of restless sleep.

9.8 Evolutionary and Social Perspective

Our ancestors lived guided by the sun. They slept at dusk and woke up at dawn.

Today, the modern world —with its screens, night shifts, and nightless cities— has generated an epidemic of circadian desynchronization.

The bipolar brain, which is genetically more sensitive, suffers in a special way from this environmental change. Restoring routines, meals at fixed times and moments of silence becomes not only medical treatment, but an act of mental ecology (Figure 8).

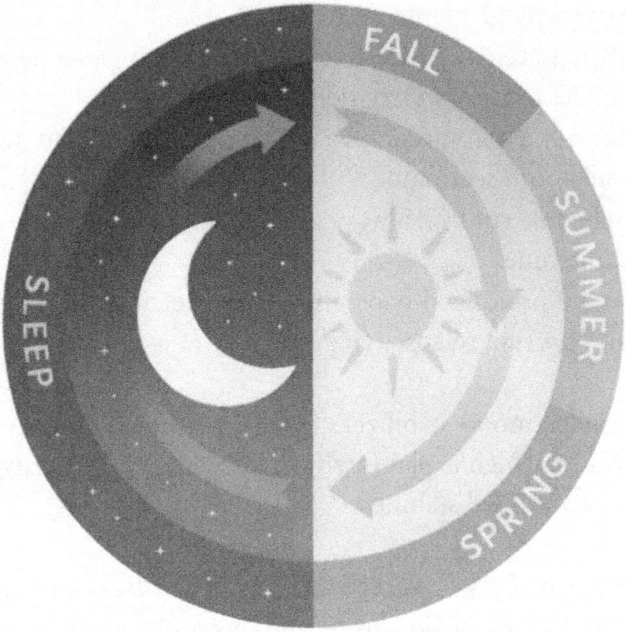

Figure 8. Conceptual representation of the circadian rhythm and sleep-wake cycle, showing the continuous alternation between day and night, light and dark, and seasonal transitions that influence mood and energy in bipolar disorder.

9.9 Prevention and Self-Care

- Get 7 to 9 hours of sleep each night.
- Do not alter rest schedules on trips or weekends.
- Avoid caffeine and alcohol after noon.
- Reduce screen use before bed.
- Increase exposure to daytime natural light.

- Consult with the psychiatrist for any prolonged changes in sleep.

Sleep is the first and most forgotten stabilizer of mood.

9.10 Synchronizing the Mind with Time

Bipolarity is not only an emotional oscillation, but also a temporal desynchronization. The body, mind, and environment should dance to the same rhythm. When one is ahead or behind, imbalance appears.

Restoring the sleep-wake cycle is more than a hygiene measure: it is a way of reconciling biology with the soul. Sleeping is the most humble and sacred act of the bipolar brain: the pause that allows the next day to begin again, with light and meaning.

CHAPTER 10
Inflammation, Neuroplasticity and Mitochondrial Dysfunction in Bipolar Disorder

When the energy of the brain turns to fire or ash.

10.1 The Brain as a Biological Field

For decades, bipolar disorder was thought to be purely chemical. Today we know that it is also cellular, immunological and metabolic. The bipolar brain not only alters its electrical communication, but also its ability to produce energy and control inflammation.

Every thought requires a biological spark: a neuron needs thousands of mitochondria to function. If those power factories fail, the mood is dull or overflowing. Thus, bipolarity can be understood as a dance between energy, inflammation and neuronal regeneration.

10.2 Inflammation as a Silent Root

Over the past two decades, numerous studies have shown that patients with bipolar disorder have elevated levels of pro-inflammatory cytokines, such as IL-6, TNF-α, and ultrasensitive CRP. These molecules, released by the immune system, alter neuronal function and modify mood circuits.

In the manic phase, the inflammatory system revs up: the body "burns" metabolically. In depression, on the other hand, it becomes slow, heavy, oxidative. Inflammation of the body becomes inflammation of thought.

10.3 Clinical Example

Claudia, 42, had been stable for a year. After a viral infection and several sleepless nights, she began to feel accelerated, overly optimistic and with grandiose thoughts.

The analyses revealed elevation of inflammatory markers. After stabilizing his sleep and treating the infection, the manic symptoms disappeared. Her case illustrates how immune processes can ignite mania or depression by affecting communication between the immune system and the brain.

10.4 Microglia: The Inflammatory Guardians of the Brain

Microglial cells are the immune system of the central nervous system. In the bipolar brain, these cells can become chronically activated, releasing cytokines that damage synaptic connections and alter neuroplasticity.

When microglia become overactive:

- Healthy synapses are destroyed.
- Increases emotional rigidity.
- Decreases cognitive flexibility.

Microglia, which should protect, end up attacking.

10.5 Neuroplasticity: the Power to Reinvent Yourself

Neuroplasticity is the brain's ability to adapt, learn, and regenerate. In bipolarity, mood swings damage that ability: connections weaken in depression and become disorganized in mania.

However, with treatment, adequate sleep, and chemical stability, the brain regains plasticity. Studies show that the neurotrophic factor BDNF (Brain-Derived Neurotrophic Factor) increases during stability and decreases in the acute phases. BDNF is like the brain's fertilizer: without it, neurons don't sprout.

Factors that increase neuroplasticity:

- Regular physical exercise.
- Cognitive and creative therapies.
- Diet rich in omega-3, magnesium and zinc.
- Restful sleep.
- Stabilizing pharmacological treatment.

Neuroplasticity shows that the bipolar brain is not doomed: it can flourish again.

10.6 Mitochondria: The Mood Energy Factories

Each neuron contains thousands of mitochondria, responsible for producing ATP, the brain's energy. In bipolar patients, the mitochondria have alterations in their DNA and enzymes: they generate less energy and more free radicals.

During mania, the mitochondria are overworked; During depression, they slow down. That cycle of "hyperenergy and exhaustion" explains why the bipolar brain alternates between euphoria and fatigue.

Drugs with beneficial mitochondrial effect

- Lithium: improves mitochondrial function and reduces oxidative stress.
- Valproic acid: increases GABA production and stabilizes energy metabolism.
- Coenzyme Q10 and omega-3: supplements that promote cellular respiration.

The treatment of the future will not only seek to balance neurotransmitters, but also to repair the brain's energy factories.

10.7 Oxidation, Stress and Neuronal Aging

Excess free radicals —unstable molecules generated by stress, alcohol, tobacco or sleep deprivation— accelerates neuronal damage. For this reason, people with untreated bipolar disorder may have premature brain aging, lower hippocampal volume, and subtle cognitive impairment.

However, the good news is that repair is possible. By stabilizing sleep, controlling stress and promoting brain oxygenation, oxidation is reduced and neuronal vitality is restored.

10.8 The Mind-Body Connection: Emotional Inflammation

Emotions also influence inflammation. Guilt, pent-up anger, and sustained frustration raise cortisol and cytokine levels, perpetuating a vicious cycle between emotional pain and immune response.

Therefore, the comprehensive approach to bipolar disorder must include body and mind: nutrition, exercise, emotional therapy and medical treatment. Well-being isn't just mental: it's immune, metabolic, and spiritual.

10.9 Therapeutic and Scientific Perspective

Modern psychiatry is moving towards a neuroimmuno-metabolic approach to bipolar disorder.

In the coming years we will see treatments that act directly on:

- Inflammatory and antioxidant genes.
- Mitochondrial stimulation.
- Regulation of the gut microbiome.
- Personalized neurotrophic therapies.

The bipolar brain is a living organism that can regenerate if given the right environment (Figure 9).

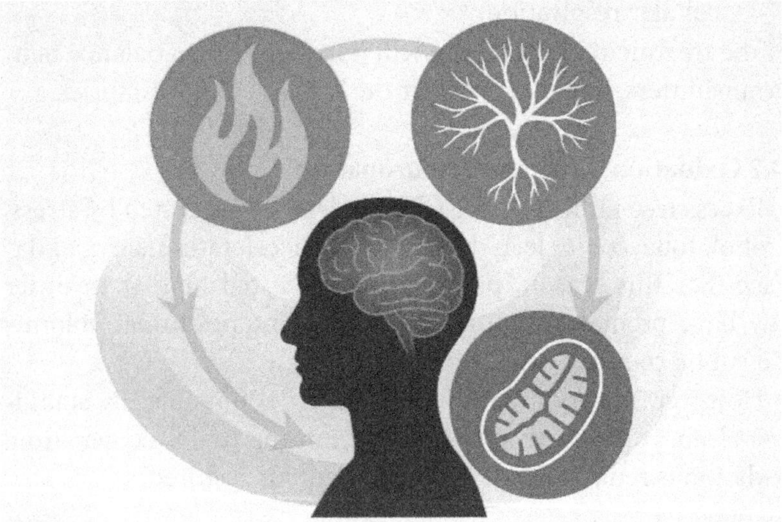

Figure 9. Conceptual representation of inflammation, neuroplasticity, and mitochondrial function in bipolar disorder. Fire symbolizes inflammation, the branching tree represents neuronal regeneration, and mitochondria embody cellular energy. Together, they reflect the balance between destruction and repair within the bipolar brain.

10.10 The Fire That Heals

Inflammation is not always an enemy: in small doses, it is a sign of repair. The dangerous thing is when it becomes chronic, silent, invisible. The bipolar brain needs to learn —like a controlled fire— to use its energy without burning out.

When the mitochondria are repaired, thinking becomes clear; When the inflammation subsides, the soul feels again without burning. Chemical balance is not a medical artifice: it is the biological way to rediscover inner peace.

CHAPTER 11
DNP-21-B Profile: Neurochemical Assessment of Bipolar

From the symptom to the circuit: the chemical map of mood.

11.1 The Neurochemical Signature of Bipolar Disorder

The DNP-21 (Dominant Neurochemical Profile–21 Questions) was designed to identify dominant patterns of neurotransmission in different psychiatric disorders.

In the case of bipolar disorder, its specific version DNP-21-B seeks to translate clinical symptoms into measurable neurochemical profiles, offering a complementary tool to traditional diagnosis.

The goal is not to replace the psychiatric interview, but to add a biological and therapeutic dimension: to understand which neurotransmitters predominate in each phase (mania, depression, or mixed state) and how to rebalance them through pharmacological, nutritional, and behavioral interventions.

11.2 The Principle of the DNP-21 Model

Each response of the instrument is associated with the functional activity of 12 neurotransmitters:

1. Dopamine.
2. Serotonin.
3. Noradrenaline.
4. GABA.
5. Glutamate.
6. Acetylcholine.
7. Histamine.
8. Endorphins.
9. Oxytocin.
10. Melatonin.

11. Cortisol.
12. Anandamide (endocannabinoid system).

The questionnaire identifies dominant patterns of excess or deficiency, which are translated into an individual neurochemical map. In bipolarity, this map usually shows dopaminergic and glutamatergic peaks during mania, and serotonergic and dopaminergic deficits in depression.

11.3 The Three Neurochemical Faces of Bipolar

a. Manic profile

- Dopamine ↑↑
- Noradrenaline ↑
- Glutamate ↑
- GABA ↓
- Variable serotonin

Clinical: euphoria, impulsivity, decreased sleep, flight of ideas, hypersexuality.

b. Depressive profile

- Dopamine ↓
- Serotonin ↓
- Noradrenaline ↓
- Cortisol ↑
- Melatonin ↓

Clinical: anhedonia, slowness, insomnia or hypersomnia, fatigue, hopelessness.

c. Mixed profile

- Dopamine ↑ / Serotonin ↓
- Glutamate ↑
- GABA ↓

Clinical: agitation with sadness, irritability, accelerated thoughts with low mood.

The DNP-21-B allows the patient to be placed on this dynamic continuum and to adjust the treatment flexibly according to the predominant phase.

11.4 Clinical Interpreting

The analysis of the questionnaire generates a neurochemical predominance index (INP) that indicates which systems require modulation.

For example:

- High dopaminergic INP → mood stabilizer with dopaminergic action (lithium, valproate, lurasidone).
- Low serotonergic INP → enhancement with lamotrigine or light therapy.
- INP GABA under → strengthening with valproate, mindfulness, and regular sleep.

In this way, the DNP-21-B translates the symptoms into a chemical language aimed at personalized intervention.

11.5 Integrative Clinical Example

Patient: Mariana, 35 years old, bipolar II.

Symptoms: Brief hypomania followed by severe fatigue and demotivation.

DNP-21-B Result:

- Dopamine ↑ in the hypomanic phase.
- Serotonin ↓ persistent.
- GABA ↓.
- Cortisol ↑ nocturnal.

Therapeutic plan:

- Lamotrigine + nocturnal quetiapine.
- Sleep hygiene and GABAergic meditation.
- Morning exercise and sun exposure.

At eight weeks, Mariana reported mood stability, increased concentration, and restorative sleep.

11.6 Clinical and Research Applications

DNP-21-B can be used in:

- Initial assessment: as a guiding map before treatment.
- Phase monitoring: to detect incipient turns.
- Clinical research: correlating neurochemical profiles with neuroimaging, genetics or inflammatory markers.

Its main value is to offer a quantifiable, dynamic and educational vision of bipolarity, helping the patient to understand their own brain (Figure 10).

11.7 Limitations and Future Projection

DNP-21-B is not a substitute for clinical judgment or diagnostic interview.

It should be integrated into medical evaluation, life history, and longitudinal observation. Its future development includes statistical validation, correlation with biomarkers and interactive digital applications (www.dnp21.com platform).

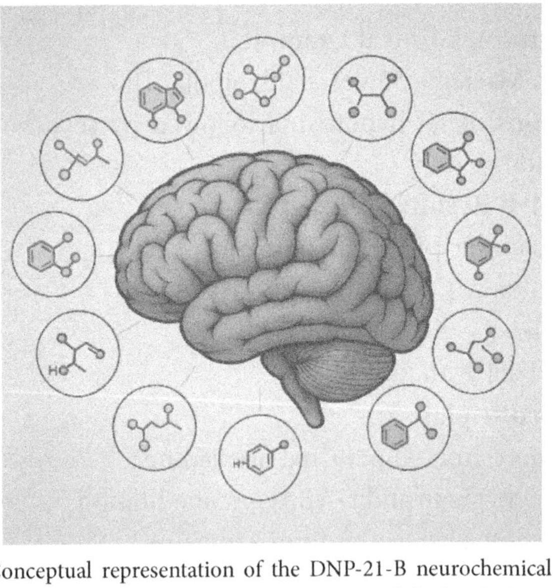

Figure 10. Conceptual representation of the DNP-21-B neurochemical map, which shows the integration of twelve neurotransmitters around the bipolar brain and symbolizes the harmony between chemistry and emotion.

11.8 The Mapping of the Mood

The DNP-21-B represents a bridge between neuroscience and everyday clinical practice. It allows us to look at bipolar disorder not as a mystery, but as a chemical map susceptible to balance.

The diagnosis ceases to be a label to become a guide: the path back to the biological and emotional center of the human being. The diagnosis is not a condemnation: it is the map that allows you to return home whenever your mood goes astray.

PART III.
Clinical Phases and Symptoms

CHAPTER 12
Manic Phase: Euphoria, Impulsivity, Hypersexuality and Delusions

When the soul burns faster than the body.

12.1 The Rise of the Storm

Mania is one of the most intense experiences that the human mind can go through. It's not just an elevated mood: it's an electrical revolution within the brain.

The patient feels that everything is possible, that every thought has meaning, that the world belongs to him. His energy seems inexhaustible, his creativity limitless, his need for sleep almost nil.

However, what begins as inspiration can transform into chaos. Mania is, in essence, an acceleration of the soul: a fire that illuminates and consumes at the same time.

12.2 The Early Signs

Before the total explosion, the body and mind emit signals:

- Decreased sleep without fatigue.
- Increased productivity or enthusiasm.
- Quick thoughts, accelerated speech.
- Extreme optimism or sudden irritability.
- Increased sociability, impulsive spending, increased sexual desire.

These signs are often mistaken for "improvement" or a high-performance stage. But the experienced psychiatrist recognizes that it is the prelude to a storm.

12.3 Manic Euphoria

Euphoria is not happiness. It is an uncontrolled expansion of the self. The patient feels capable of anything; his ideas flow with dazzling speed. In the brain, dopamine and glutamate spike, while GABA and serotonin drop.

Clinical case

Daniel, 34, consulted after spending his savings on an alleged "millionaire investment". He had slept two hours a night, wrote endless projects and felt "the mission to change the country". He firmly believed in his genius, without perceiving the risks. Mania turns confidence into omnipotence and energy into insomnia.

12.4 Impulsivity and Loss of Judgment

The prefrontal brake system, which regulates behavior, weakens during mania. Decisions become immediate, without reflection.

The patient acts according to what he feels, not according to what is convenient.

Common behaviors:

- Excessive expenses or indebtedness.
- Risky sexual behaviors.
- Great projects without planning.
- Verbal or physical aggressiveness in the face of frustrations.

It is not a question of moral irresponsibility, but of a neurochemical disconnection between impulse and consciousness.

12.5 Hypersexuality and Overflowing Desire

Hypersexuality is a frequent and often embarrassing symptom. The patient feels intensely desired and desiring; his libido multiplies. This is due to the increase in dopamine, testosterone and norepinephrine.

Clinical case

Marta, 29, said: "I felt that I could conquer anyone. It was a physical need, as if my body demanded contact from me". Then, in the depressive phase, the predominant feeling was guilt. Manic hypersexuality is not a vice: it is a biochemical alteration of perception and desire.

12.6 Verbiage and Racing Thinking

The manic patient's language flows without pause. Speak quickly, change the subject, invent neologisms or rhymes. Often the psychiatrist must interrupt you to redirect the conversation.

This mental acceleration is known as idea flight. The brain processes associations so quickly that it loses external coherence. At the neural level, a temporal hyperconnection is observed: many networks activated simultaneously.

12.7 Irritability and Aggressiveness

Not all manias are joyful. Some patients present with dysphoric mania, with a predominance of irritability, anger, and tension. Euphoria is mixed with intolerance, especially towards those who try to set limits.

The family environment is often exhausted: arguments, breakdown of relationships, loss of work. Therefore, early detection of this subtype is essential to avoid acute crises or hospitalizations.

12.8 Delusions and Psychotic Symptoms

In extreme phases, the mind crosses the boundary of reality. Delusions of grandeur, power, or divine inspiration may arise. The patient may believe that he has a cosmic mission or that he receives messages from the universe.

Example

Ana, 37, arrived at the hospital claiming that she could "talk to the stars". He hadn't slept for six days, wrote messages to public figures and talked nonstop. After stabilization with lithium and antipsychotic, he regained his sanity and acknowledged the nature of his episode. Mania is, in a way, a lucid dream where the imagination is emancipated from rational control.

12.9 Neurobiology of Mania

- Dopamine ↑↑ → hyperactivity, pleasure, creativity.
- Glutamate ↑ → Accelerated Thinking.
- Noradrenaline ↑ → energy and constant alertness.
- GABA ↓ → loss of cortical brake.
- Variable serotonin → oscillations between euphoria and irritability.

This chemical storm explains both the momentary genius and the subsequent collapse.

12.10 Consequences and Cumulative Damage

Each untreated manic episode leaves neural fingerprints. Connections are weakened, sleep is disturbed, and emotional thresholds are lowered.

In addition, euphoria is often followed by an abrupt descent into depression or total exhaustion. Therefore, the goal of treatment is not only to "control the crisis", but to protect the brain from future relapse.

12.11 Therapeutic Strategy

- Lithium: classic stabilizer, effective in prevention.
- Valproate and carbamazepine: reduce impulsivity and arousal.
- Atypical antipsychotics: quetiapine, olanzapine, risperidone, lurasidone.
- Sleep control: melatonin, circadian hygiene, hospitalization if necessary.
- Family psychoeducation: detect signs of relapse.

Treatment does not shut down creativity, but protects the mind so that creativity does not turn into destruction.

12.12 The Light That Blinds

Mania is the fire that reveals human potential and at the same time its fragility. It is the brain's attempt to live beyond its biological limits. The psychiatrist must accompany this fire with respect, without extinguishing it or letting it consume the patient.

The goal is not to silence the mind, but to teach it to sustain its own intensity without losing its balance (Figure 11).

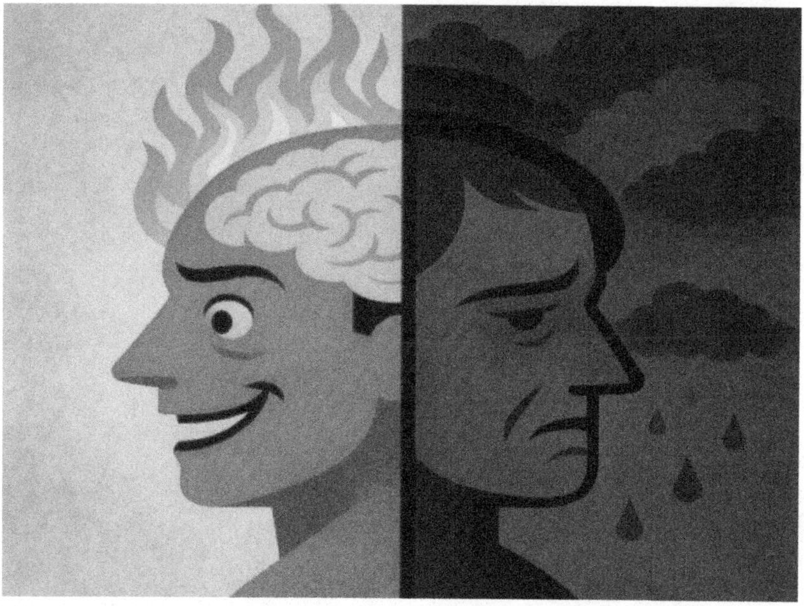

Figure 11. Conceptual representation of the manic phase in bipolar disorder. The image contrasts the brightness and energy of mania with the latent risk of chaos and collapse, symbolizing the brain's struggle between enlightenment and control.

CHAPTER 13
Depressive Phase: Hopelessness, Mental Slowness and Suicidal Risk

When the mind shuts down and the soul loses color.

13.1 The Silent Descent

After the vertigo of mania, emptiness arrives. Bipolar depression is not simple sadness; It is a total deactivation of the nervous system. The brain that once burned with ideas now becomes heavy, slow, without energy.

The patient feels that every thought is difficult, that the body weighs more than it can sustain. Unlike unipolar depression, bipolar depression is usually deeper, more abrupt, and often accompanied by guilt, extreme fatigue, and suicidal ideation.

It is not weakness or lack of will: it is a biochemical fall that robs the ability to feel pleasure and hope.

13.2 The Slowness of Thought

In depression, mental processing slows down. Simple tasks seem like mountains, conversations become effort. The patient describes his mind as "cloudy", "slow", or "empty".

Neuroimaging shows hypoactivity in the dorsolateral prefrontal cortex and basal ganglia, as well as decreased blood flow in the hippocampus. In clinical terms, this translates into indecision, low concentration and difficulty planning. Depression is the brain trying to save energy because it feels like life doesn't deserve it.

13.3 Anhedonia: Offline Pleasure

One of the most characteristic symptoms is anhedonia, the inability to enjoy what used to generate pleasure. It is not about sadness, but about disconnection.

The dopaminergic system —especially the nucleus accumbens— shuts down, leaving the patient emotionally anesthetized. Coffee doesn't taste the same, music doesn't excite, hugs don't console. The world becomes flat, without affective texture.

In depression, the mind doesn't want to die: it just wants to stop feeling.

13.4 Fatigue, Sleep and Altered Circadian Rhythm

The depressed bipolar patient may sleep too much or not at all. Both alterations are an expression of the same dysfunctional axis between the hypothalamus, melatonin and cortisol.

The body enters a kind of frustrated hibernation: it needs to rest, but rest does not repair. Many refer to an existential fatigue: a tiredness of the soul rather than of the body.

13.5 Guilt, Self-Criticism and Hopelessness

Bipolar depression has a moral tone: the patient feels guilty for no reason. He believes that he has failed his family, his purpose, God. This type of ruminative thinking is associated with hyperactivity of the medial prefrontal section and low serotonin.

The internal discourse becomes cruel: "I'm good for nothing", "I ruined my life", "I'd be better off dead". These phrases are not rational thoughts: they are the chemical echo of an inflamed brain without energy.

13.6 Suicidal Risk

Among all psychiatric disorders, bipolar disorder has the highest risk of suicide: up to 20% of patients attempt suicide at some point.

The risk increases in mixed periods, where energy returns before hope. The psychiatrist should directly explore suicidal ideation, bluntly:

- "Have you thought about dying?"
- "Have you imagined how I would do it?"
- "Have you made any plans?"

Asking doesn't induce the idea: it saves lives.

13.7 The Depressive Body

The body also suffers:

- Muscle pain or headaches.
- Digestive or immune problems.
- Changes in appetite and weight.
- Feeling of internal cold.

Depression doesn't just affect the brain; It is a systemic disorder, with endocrine, immune and mitochondrial alterations.

13.8 Differences with Unipolar Depression

Table 2 summarizes the main clinical differences between bipolar depression and unipolar depression, highlighting onset patterns, variations in energy and sleep, family history, and differential response to antidepressants, fundamental aspects for a correct diagnosis and prevention of therapeutic errors.

Table 2. Key Clinical Differences Between Bipolar Depression and Unipolar Depression

Appearance	Bipolar	Unipolar
Home	More abrupt	Progressive
Energy	Alternates between fatigue and agitation	Constant fatigue
Sleep	More variable	More predictable
Family History	High presence of bipolarity	Lower incidence
Response to anti-depressants	Risk of manic swerving	Generally favorable

That is why it is essential not to diagnose as "major depression" what is actually covert bipolarity.

13.9 Therapeutic Strategies

a. Pharmacological

- Lamotrigine: ideal stabilizer for bipolar depression.
- Quetiapine and lurasidone: antipsychotics with antidepressant effect.
- Avoid SSRIs alone: they can induce mania.
- Lithium: reduces suicide risk and improves neuroprotection.

b. Non-pharmacological

- Bipolar cognitive-behavioral therapy.
- Interpersonal and social rhythm therapy.
- Morning phototherapy.
- Regular physical exercise.
- Stable daily routine and restful sleep.

Clinical example

Carlos, 46, had overcome a manic phase six months earlier. Now he barely got out of bed, he said he felt "empty". When DNP-21-B was applied, a severe depressive profile was observed (dopamine ↓, serotonin ↓, GABA ↑). Treatment with lamotrigine, psychotherapy, and exposure to morning light were adjusted.

Three months later, Carlos resumed his work, his readings and smiled again when talking about his children. The depression hadn't completely disappeared, but he'd learned not to identify with it.

13.10 The Winter of the Mind

Bipolar depression is a cerebral winter: necessary, painful, and sometimes restorative. Treatment is not just about "lifting your spirits", but about rebuilding energy, identity, and hope.

The depressed soul is not broken: it is hibernating, waiting for the return of the light. And each time that light returns, it does so with a new depth: the realization that even the silence of the mind is part of the cycle of mental life (Figure 12).

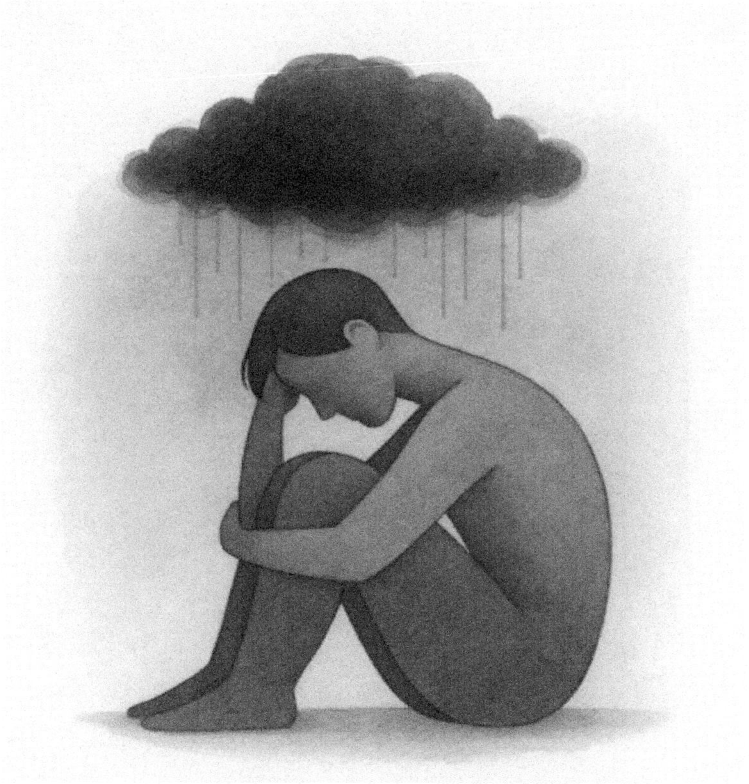

Figure 12. Conceptual representation of the depressive phase in bipolar disorder. The image portrays deep sadness and isolation under a dark cloud, symbolizing the heavy burden of hopelessness.

CHAPTER 14
Mixed Episodes: when the Body Runs but the Soul Cries

The inner storm of the bipolar brain.

14.1 Two Storms in the Same Sky

Mixed episodes are the most painful paradox of bipolar disorder. The patient feels a manic energy in the body, but a depressive hopelessness in the soul.

His mind is racing, but his motivation is destroyed. He can laugh and cry in the same minute, plan grandiose projects while contemplating the idea of suicide. The mixture of opposing symptoms —simultaneous manic and depressive— creates a state of extreme suffering and confusion for the patient and his or her environment.

14.2 What Happens in the Brain during a Mixed Episode?

In neuroimaging, simultaneous spikes in dopamine and glutamate are observed, combined with a drop in serotonin and GABA. In other words, the brain is excited and depressed at the same time.

This combination produces:

- Racing but negative thoughts.
- High energy with hopelessness.
- Impulsivity with guilt.
- Irritability with fatigue.

The limbic system is hyperactivated, while the prefrontal cortex (which regulates emotions) is exhausted. The result is an overflowing and directionless mind.

Clinical example

Andrea, 32 years old, went to the emergency room saying: "I can't stop thinking, but everything I think is horrible". He spoke fast, did not sleep, had lost weight and cried easily. She alternated between euphoria and tears, between life projects and suicidal thoughts.

DNP-21-B revealed dopaminergic and glutamatergic hyperactivity with serotonergic deficiency. After starting treatment with valproate, quetiapine and intensive psychotherapy, his mind began to slow down. "I feel like the noise went down", she said at three weeks.

14.3 Typical Symptoms of the Mixed Episode

Table 3 illustrates the relationship between the frequent clinical symptoms of mood disorders, their subjective and behavioral manifestations, and the main neurochemical systems involved. The purpose of this table is to facilitate an integrative understanding between clinical phenomenology and neurobiology.

Table 3. Correlation between affective symptoms, clinical manifestations and neurochemical systems involved

Type of symptom	Clinical example	Neurotransmitter involved
Angry euphoria	"Everything bothers me, but I can't stop".	Dopamine ↑ + GABA ↓
Accelerated and negative thinking	"I think a thousand bad things a minute".	Glutamate ↑ + Serotonin ↓
Physical agitation with emotional fatigue	Restlessness, insomnia, crying	Noradrenaline ↑ + Cortisol ↑
Impulsive behaviors with subsequent guilt	Risky spending or sexuality	Dopamine ↑ + Serotonin ↓
High suicide risk	Enough energy to act	Dopamine ↑ + Serotonin ↓ + GABA ↓

14.5 The Highest Risk: Hopeless Energy

In pure depression, the person does not have the strength to act. In pure mania, the energy is usually positive. But in the mixed episode, the patient has enough energy to carry out suicidal impulses without being stopped by the pain.

For this reason, these episodes are considered psychiatric emergencies. Sleep control and immediate pharmacological containment can save lives.

14.6 Differential Diagnosis

Mixed episodes may be confused with:

- Borderline personality disorder (due to emotional instability).
- ADHD (due to impulsivity and agitation).
- Generalized anxiety (due to mental hyperactivity).

However, the cyclical pattern and family history of bipolar are key to accurate diagnosis.

14.7 Therapeutic Management

a. Pharmacological

- Sodium valproate: of choice in mixed episodes.
- Carbamazepine: useful in irritability and aggressiveness.
- Atypical antipsychotics: quetiapine, olanzapine or lurasidone.
- Avoid antidepressants: They can worsen arousal or suicidal risk.

b. Non-pharmacological

- Sleep control and reduction of sensory stimuli.
- Emotional containment psychotherapy.
- Family education to recognize early signs.
- Gentle exercise and structured routine.

The treatment seeks to slow down the brain without shutting it down.

14.8 Subjective Experience

Many patients describe the mixed episode as "having an engine running in a dark room". They can't stop their thoughts, but they also can't find meaning in them. Pain is physical, psychic and existential at the same time. The body wants to run, but the soul wants to disappear. Empathic accompaniment and psychiatric containment are essential (Figure 13).

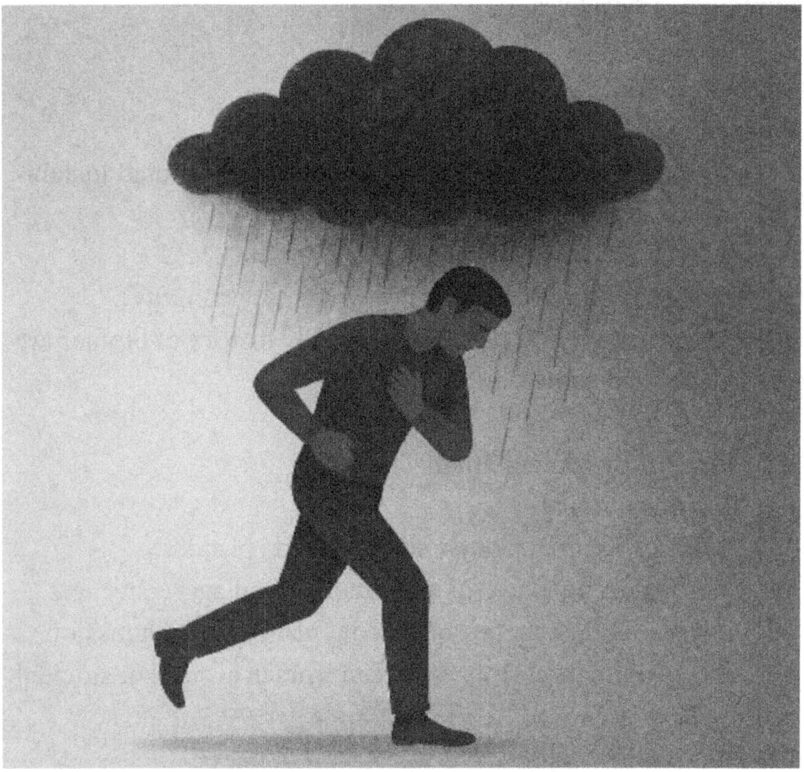

Figure 13. Conceptual representation of mixed episodes in bipolar disorder. The figure running under a storm cloud symbolizes the paradox of simultaneous turmoil and hopelessness: when the body moves with manic speed, but the heart is oppressed by depression.

14.9 Recovery and Follow-up

Exiting a mixed episode requires patience. Circadian rhythms and neurotransmitters need weeks to stabilize. Once stability is achieved, it is key to reinforce prevention: regular sleep, DNP-21-B monitoring, psychotherapy and constant pharmacological control.

Each recovery strengthens the patient's awareness of his mind: he learns to recognize small imbalances before they become storms.

14.10 Lightning and Shadow

Mixed episodes are at the heart of bipolarity: the coexistence of life and death, light and darkness, energy and hopelessness. The psychiatrist not only treats an illness, but a mind that tries to survive its own contradictions. When the body runs and the soul cries, the art of psychiatry is to accompany that race until both walk together again.

CHAPTER 15
Hypomania: Energy Disguised as Success

The brightness that precedes the storm.

15.1 The Most Deceptive Phase of Bipolar Disorder

Hypomania is the most subtle and tempting form of bipolar disorder. There are no delusions or total lack of control, and that is why it goes unnoticed by many patients, families and even professionals.

The individual feels better than ever: more productive, more sociable, more creative, more self-confident. But beneath that apparent perfection hides a neurochemical acceleration that, without treatment, can turn into a manic storm or a depressive fall. Hypomania is not equilibrium: it is the bright edge of imbalance.

15.2 The Functional Face of Hypomania

Many patients say, "I wish I could stay this way all the time". And it's understandable. During hypomania:

- Thought flows quickly, but logically.
- Sleep decreases, but the body does not become fatigued.
- Creativity intensifies.
- The conversation is fluid and charismatic.
- Sexual desire increases.
- The mood is optimistic and expansive.

This superior performance generates positive reinforcement from the environment: praise, promotions, recognition. The patient is convinced that he is "cured" or "at his best".

15.3 Neurobiology of Hypomania

During hypomania, there is a moderate increase in dopamine and glutamate, with a slight decrease in GABA. The limbic system is activated, but the prefrontal cortex still manages to maintain relative control.

This combination creates a state of mental hyperclarity without perceptual distortion.

The brain feels "in focus", but it's actually on the verge of overload. It's the neurochemical equivalent of driving a car at 160 km/h on a straight highway: the trip seems perfect... until a curve appears.

Clinical example

Lucía, 28 years old, a journalist, described her hypomania as follows: "It was as if everything made sense. I woke up with energy, I wrote articles in hours, I talked to everyone. But then, when I couldn't sleep, I started to feel like my head wouldn't stop".

In their case, DNP-21-B showed a high dopaminergic profile and low GABA. Early intervention with mood stabilizer prevented the episode from progressing to full-blown mania.

15.4 Differences between Hypomania and Mania

Table 4 compares the fundamental clinical features of hypomania and mania. Differences in energy level, sleep, judgment, social behavior, need for hospitalization and duration of episodes are also highlighted, key elements for an adequate diagnostic evaluation and therapeutic decision-making.

Table 4. Clinical differences between hypomania and mania

Feature	Hypomania	Mania
Energy Level	Augmented	Extremely high
Sleep	Decreased without fatigue	Total insomnia
Trial	Partially preserved	Severely affected
Social behavior	Charismatic and productive	Impulsive, disruptive
Need for hospitalization	Not usual	Frequent
Duration	≥4 days	≥7 days

For this reason, many patients with bipolar II go years without diagnosis, believing that they are simply "high-energy" people.

15.5 The Risk of False Well-Being

The problem with hypomania is its clinical invisibility. The patient does not seek help because he feels good, and the environment reinforces his behavior. But that excess activity, if left unregulated, fatigues the dopaminergic and circadian circuits, setting the stage for a depressive fall. In bipolarity, any unstabilized ascent ends in a fall.

15.6 Creative Hypomania versus Destructive Hypomania

Not all hypomania is negative. In its mild phase, it can enhance artistic, intellectual or professional productivity. However, when it is prolonged, risky behaviors appear: unnecessary expenses, interpersonal conflicts, work hyperactivity. The therapeutic challenge is not to eliminate the energy, but to channel it without it overflowing.

15.7 Clinical Approach

a. Pharmacological

- Lithium or lamotrigine: regulate excitability without sedation.
- Quetiapine or lurasidone: stabilize mood and sleep.
- Avoid stimulants or antidepressants: they can precipitate mania.

b. Psychological

- Psychoeducation: teaching to recognize early signs.
- Social rhythm therapy: reinforce schedules and rest.
- Mindfulness or breathing techniques: to slow down the mind.

c. Behavioral

- Set realistic limits to the activity.
- Reduce multitasking.
- Avoid impulsive financial or emotional decisions.

15.8 Hypomania in Art and Science

Many creative geniuses have lived on this threshold: Van Gogh, Newton, Virginia Woolf, Beethoven. During their hypomanic phases, they produced immortal works; during depressive periods, they isolated themselves or collapsed.

The history of humanity is full of bipolar minds that shone excessively and were extinguished prematurely. The modern goal of psychiatry is not to eliminate that light, but to help the patient sustain it without getting burned.

15.9 The Mirage of Equilibrium

Hypomania is the most dangerous phase because it is mistaken for success. It is the moment when the patient feels invincible just before losing control.

The psychiatrist must help him recognize that not all euphoria is health, and that true well-being does not depend on intensity, but on balance. Hypomania is the mirage where the brain believes it has found perfection (Figure 14).

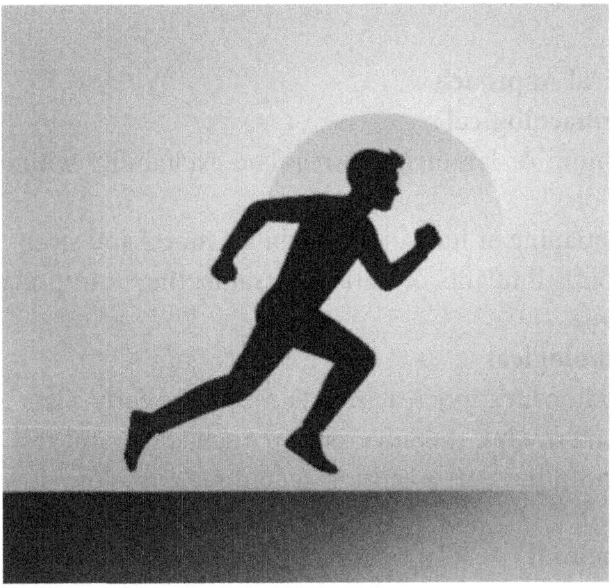

Figure 14. Conceptual representation of hypomania in bipolar disorder. The image symbolizes the impulse of energy and confidence that propels the individual forward, illuminated by enthusiasm but with the latent shadow of imbalance.

CHAPTER 16
Psychotic Symptoms in Extreme Phases

When emotion becomes perception.

16.1 The Mind That Overflows Reality

In the most intense episodes of bipolarity —whether manic or depressive— the brain can exceed the limits of normal perception and generate psychotic symptoms.

It is not "madness" in the popular sense, but an emotional amplification so powerful that the thought is distorted.

The patient does not imagine random things: his delusions and hallucinations are usually symbolic extensions of his affective state. That is why bipolar psychopathology is different from schizophrenia: in bipolarity, delirium has emotional roots.

16.2 The Boundary Between Emotion and Perception

The human brain translates feelings into interpretations of the environment. When the limbic system (amygdala, hippocampus, orbitofrontal cortex) becomes overactive, intense emotions can alter perception.

In mania, the world is perceived as expansive and full of divine signs. In depression, everything seems hostile or empty. Bipolar psychosis is, in essence, a metaphor for the internal state projected outwards. One does not see what is, but what the spirit allows one to see.

16.3 Types of Psychotic Symptoms in Bipolar Disorder

Table 5 describes the main psychotic symptoms associated with bipolar disorder, differentiating them according to their phenomenological content and the mood phase in which they predominate, which is essential for differential diagnosis, severity assessment, and therapeutic planning.

Table 5. Psychotic symptoms in bipolar disorder according to mood phase

Type	Description	Predominant phase
Delusions of grandeur	Beliefs of power, mission or special destiny.	Mania
Congruent auditory hallucinations	Voices that encourage or confirm expansive ideas.	Mania
Delusions of guilt or ruin	Belief that you have caused a catastrophe or are guilty of everything.	Depression
Accusatory auditory hallucinations	Voices that insult or criticize.	Depression
Religious delusions	Intense mystical experiences, "conversations with God".	Both phases
Somatic delusions	Feeling like the body is rotting, burning, or disappearing.	Severe depression

These symptoms are congruent with mood: the content of the delirium reflects the dominant emotion.

Clinical example of mystical mania

Rafael, 41 years old, art teacher. He was taken to the hospital after three sleepless nights. He said that the universe spoke to him through colors and that he should "save the world with a mural of light".

He spoke fervently, convinced of his divine mission. After stabilization with lithium and atypical antipsychotic, he regained lucidity. A few weeks later he said: "It was as if everything made sense... but it was too much". His delirium was an artistic expression of his euphoria, not a primary psychotic break.

Clinical Example of Delusional Depression

Elena, 56 years old, mother of three children. She was hospitalized for refusing to eat. He said, "I don't deserve to be fed. God punishes me for failing". He showed extreme guilt and religious delusions congruent with his deep sadness.

His treatment combined antipsychotic (quetiapine), stabilizer (lamotrigine) and compassionate psychotherapy. After two months, his faith was transformed: "I still believe in God, but I don't think he hates me anymore.

16.4 Neurobiology of Bipolar Psychosis

During psychotic episodes, the following is observed:

1. Dopaminergic hyperactivity in the mesolimbic pathway (delusions and hallucinations).
2. Hypofrontality (less rational control).
3. Circadian desynchronization (loss of sleep-wake rhythm).
4. Neuroimmune inflammation and glutamatergic dysfunction.

The combination creates a state where the imagination becomes sensory real. The patient does not "invent": his brain experiences emotion as concrete perception.

16.5 Treatment

a. Pharmacological

- Atypical antipsychotics: quetiapine, olanzapine, risperidone, lurasidone.
- Mood stabilizers: lithium, valproate, lamotrigine.
- Avoid antidepressants alone: they can aggravate psychosis.
- Regular sleep and circadian rhythm.

b. Psychological and spiritual

- Supportive psychotherapy: reality reconstruction.
- Symbolic integration: reinterpreting the mystical or delusional experience in a healthy way.

- Family accompaniment: avoid judgments or direct confrontations.

The goal is not to deny the experience, but togive it back a human and therapeutic meaning.

16.6 Differences with Schizophrenia

Table 6 offers a comparison of the fundamental clinical characteristics of bipolar psychosis and schizophrenia, highlighting the differences in the pattern of onset, delusional content, temporal evolution, affectivity and response to treatment, key elements for differential diagnosis and appropriate therapeutic selection.

Table 6. Clinical differences between bipolar psychosis and schizophrenia

Feature	Bipolar psychosis	Schizophrenia
Home	Episodic and mood-associated	Chronic and progressive
Content of delirium	Congruent with emotion	Incongruent or bizarre
Recovery between episodes	Complete	Partial
Affectivity	Intense and variable	Flattened
Lithium Response	Good	Limited

The bipolar patient with psychosis regains his original identity once the chemical storm dissipates.

16.7 Humanistic Perspective

The psychotic phases of bipolar are not only a loss of reason, but an extreme language of the soul. They are the brain's attempt to translate unbearable emotions into images and symbols.

For this reason, compassionate treatment is essential: it is not only about medicating, but about helping the patient to integrate what they have experienced. Psychosis does not always destroy; sometimes, he reveals.

16.8 The Mind that Saw Too Much

Psychotic symptoms in bipolar disorder are the final boundary between emotion and perception, between the human and the transcendent. The psychiatrist's challenge is to accompany this journey without judging it, helping to transform delirium into understanding.

The bipolar brain, when it overflows, does not seek madness: it seeks meaning. And when calm comes, the mind remembers that even excess reality can heal if it is given a name and a place within one's personal history (Figure 15).

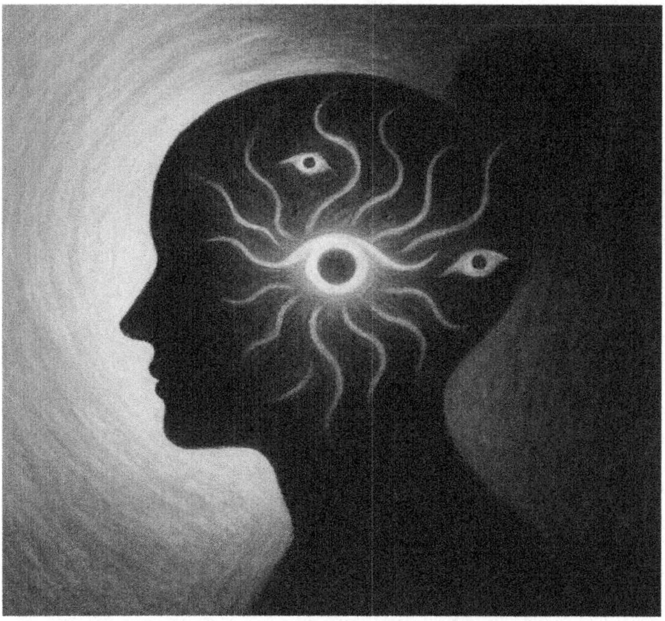

Figure 15. Conceptual representation of psychotic symptoms in bipolar disorder. The luminous eye inside the head symbolizes perception turned inwards: when emotion overwhelms reason and the mind begins to see its own feelings as reality.

PART IV. Diagnosis and Evaluation

CHAPTER 17
Psychiatric Interview Focused on the Bipolar Spectrum

The art of listening to the rhythms of the mood.

17.1 Diagnosing Movement, Not Timing

Bipolar disorder is not diagnosed with a photo: it is diagnosed with a film. It is not enough to observe how a person feels today; you have to understand how their mood has oscillated over time.

The psychiatric interview focused on the bipolar spectrum seeks to capture those subtle changes: the periods of acceleration, the pauses, the silences and the falls. To diagnose bipolarity is to listen to the inner music of the mood —its crescendos, its pauses, and its dissonances.

17.2 The Importance of the Vital Context

Before talking about symptoms, the psychiatrist must know the patient's biographical history:

- Stages of life with increased energy or sadness.
- Sudden changes in relationships, jobs or habits.
- Use of substances or stimulants.
- Family history of bipolar, depression, or suicide.
- Cultural and religious factors that shape the perception of mood.

Bipolarity does not arise in a vacuum; it is a dance between genetics, environment and meaning.

17.3 Clinical Dialogue

A good interview is not an interrogation; it is a conversation aimed at understanding the pattern.

Some key questions are:

- "Have you had times when you slept little, but felt full of energy?"
- "Have you felt like your mind doesn't stop and that anything seems possible?"
- "Have you gone from feeling elated to deeply sad in a few days?"
- "Has anyone in your family had severe mood swings or lithium treatments?"

These questions make it possible to detect cyclicity and distinguish it from unipolar or personality disorders.

17.4 Phases as Emotional Language

Bipolar mood is not only a biological alteration, but also an emotional language. Each phase expresses something different. Table 7 presents the relationship between the emotional language expressed by the patient and the underlying psychological needs in each phase of bipolar disorder, which offers a clinical tool to improve therapeutic empathy and guide interventions more adjusted to the predominant emotional state.

Table 7. Emotional language and psychological needs according to the phase of bipolar disorder

Phase	Emotional language	Underlying Need
Mania	"I can do anything".	Control, power, recognition
Hypomania	"I'm the best version of myself".	Validation, creativity
Depression	"Nothing makes sense".	Affection, comfort
Mixed episode	"I can't stop, but I want to disappear".	Containment, calm

When the clinician understands this language, he stops seeing symptoms and begins to hear meanings.

17.5 Behavioral and Nonverbal Observation

The bipolar diagnosis is also perceived in the body and tone:

- Changes in speech rate.
- Body posture (upright and expansive versus hunched over and slow).
- Shiny or unkempt clothing.
- Variable eye contact.
- Broad gesticulation in mania; immobility in depression.

The psychiatrist observes respectfully, without labeling, looking for the rhythm behind the gesture.

17.6 Use of DNP-21-B as an Integrative Tool

The dominant neurochemical profile (DNP-21-B) complements the clinical interview by identifying patterns of dominant or deficient neurotransmitters. It makes it possible to distinguish, for example, whether a depressive patient has a low dopaminergic component or an excess of glutamate, which guides treatment.

Example:

- High dopamine + low GABA → risk of hypomania.
- Low serotonin + low norepinephrine → pure depression.
- High glutamate + high dopamine → mixed episodes.

The modern psychiatric interview unites the word with biology.

17.7 Suicidal and Functional Risk Assessment

Every diagnosis must include an assessment of the vital and functional risk:

- Thoughts of death or hopelessness.
- Self-destructive impulses.
- Work, academic or family injuries.
- Substance abuse.

The goal is not just to classify, but to protect. The interview does not seek a diagnosis, it seeks an opportunity for prevention.

17.8 Common Diagnostic Difficulties

Bipolar disorder is often confused with:

- Unipolar depression (when only one phase is seen).
- Borderline personality disorder (due to emotional impulsivity).
- ADHD (due to restlessness and distraction).
- Generalized anxiety (due to mental hyperactivity).

That's why the interview should include the mood timeline —a complete emotional timeline— (Figure 16).

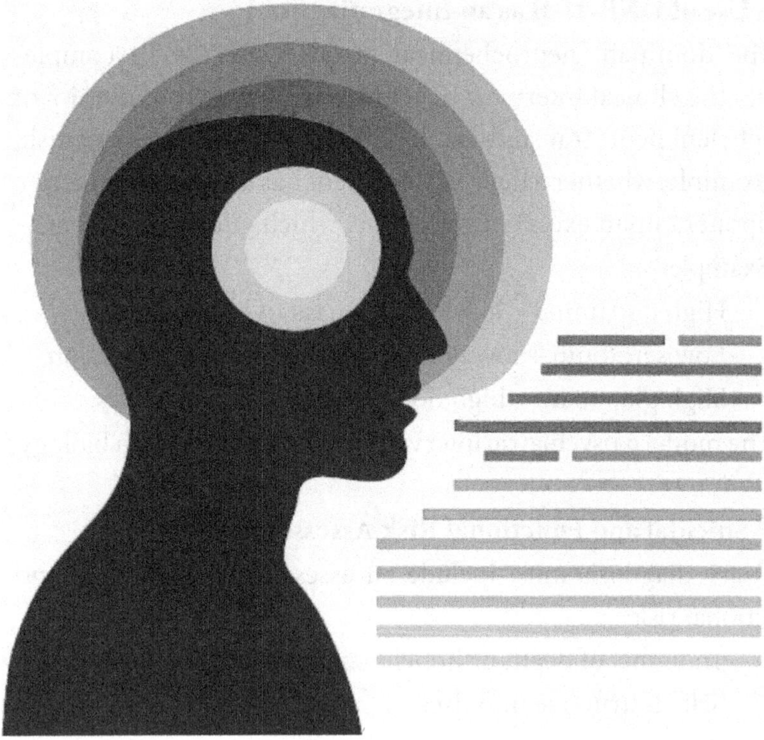

Figure 16. Conceptual representation of the psychiatric interview focused on the bipolar spectrum. The image symbolizes empathy, listening, and the flow of understanding between clinician and patient, where dialogue becomes the bridge between biology and meaning.

17.9 The Art of Rapport

The bipolar patient is sensitive, perceptive, and has often been judged or misdiagnosed. The psychiatrist must create a safe space where the patient can speak without fear of losing their dignity.

True rapport (fluid communication) is achieved when the patient feels that the clinician understands his rhythm without trying to dominate it. To listen to the bipolar is to listen to a soul that has traveled from the sun to the night and still seeks its dawn.

17.10 Diagnosing with Empathy and Science

The interview focused on the bipolar spectrum is not a questionnaire; it is a human encounter. It involves science, intuition, and respect for the patient's emotional complexity. A good diagnosis does not label: it reveals a map.

And every map, well read, leads back home. The diagnosis is not a condemnation: it is the map that allows you to return home whenever your mood goes astray.

CHAPTER 18
DNP-21-B Diagnostic Scales and Neurochemical Profile

Quantify what you feel, understand what you measure.

18.1 When Emotion Translates into Numbers

In psychiatry, measuring does not mean reducing human complexity to numbers, buttranslating suffering into a language that science can hear. The diagnostic scales and the DNP-21-B model (dominant neurochemical profile; The Dominant Neurochemical Profile are two sides of the same map: one quantifies behavior; the other reveals its neurochemical root).

The scale measures the phenomenon; DNP-21-B explains its biology. The use of both together allows for a more accurate, more humane and more personalized diagnosis.

18.2 Measuring Euphoria

The Young's Mania Scale (YMRS) assesses the intensity of the manic phase. It includes 11 items that qualify from expansive humor to impaired judgment.

Score:

- 0-12 = normal or mild hypomania.
- 13-19 = moderate hypomania.
- 20-40 = clinically significant mania.

Clinical interpretation:

- Increased energy, speed of thought, insomnia, grandiosity.

DNP-21-B neurochemical mapping:

- Dopamine ↑↑
- Glutamate ↑
- GABA ↓
- Serotonin ↓ or normal

Example:

A patient with YMRS = 28 shows hyperactivity, rapid speech, and multiple plans.

DNP-21-B reveals dopaminergic-glutamatergic predominance: confirmed diagnosis of acute manic phase. Each dot in the YMRS is an echo of accelerated synapses.

18.3 Detecting the Hidden Spectrum

The MDQ (Mood Disorder Questionnaire) helps identify undiagnosed bipolar disorder in patients presenting with depression. It consists of 13 items on euphoria, irritability, activity and sleep reduction.

Resultado positivo:

- 7 or more affirmative answers + simultaneous occurrence.

Clinical interpretation:

- Detects a history of unnoticed hypomanic episodes.

DNP-21-B correspondence:

- Oscillations of dopamine, norepinephrine and serotonin in cyclical patterns.
- You may anticipate risk of paradoxical response to antidepressants.

Example:

Patient with recurrent depression and MDQ positive → DNP-21-B profile. Shows unstable dopamine. Diagnosis was adjusted to type II bipolarity and inappropriate antidepressant treatment was avoided.

18.4 Functional Brightness

The HCL-32 Hypomania Symptom Checklist explores mild hypomanic episodes, characteristic of bipolar II and intermediate spectra. It evaluates 32 statements about behavior, energy, sleep, creativity and sociability.

Score:

- ≥ 14 = probable hypomania.
- 10-13 = high energy trait without pathologies.
- < 10 = normal rank.

DNP-21-B Neurochemical Interpretation:

- Dopamine ↑ moderate.
- GABA ↓ mild.
- Stable or slightly low serotonin.

Example:

A designer with 16 points refers to productivity, charisma and little sleep. The DNP-21-B confirms hypomanic dopaminergic pattern: balance achieved with lamotrigine and sleep regulation.

18.5 The Clinician's Gaze

The CGI-BP Clinical Global Impression Scale for Bipolar Disorder integrates the psychiatrist's expertise.

Evaluate:

- Severity of the current episode.
- Overall improvement after treatment.
- Therapeutic efficacy.

Escale: 1 = normal → 7 = extremely sick.

Example:

Patient with severe mania (CGI-BP = 6) improves to CGI-BP = 2 after eight weeks on lithium.

Relation to DNP-21-B:

- Monitoring the neurochemical profile in parallel shows reduction in dopamine and glutamate, compensatory increase in GABA, → biological confirmation of improvement.

The CGI-BP measures music; the DNP-21-B shows which instruments were retuned.

18.6 The Neurochemical Map of the Bipolar Spectrum

The DNP-21-B 21-question questionnaire is a tool created to identify the dominant neurotransmitter profile in each patient with bipolar disorder. Unlike traditional scales, it does not only evaluate symptoms, but also the biochemical signature that originates them.

Main axes:

- Dopamine: motivation, energy, impulsivity.
- Serotonin: calm, sleep, emotional regulation.

- Noradrenaline: alertness, attention, stress.
- GABA: corticalbrake, stability.
- Glutamate: excitation, plasticity.
- Acetylcholine, oxytocin, endorphins, histamine, melatonin, anandamide and cortisol complete the map of 12 neurotransmitters (Table 8).

Table 8. Typical bipolar DNP-21-B profile

Phase	Dominant neurotransmitters	Signature pattern
Mania	Dopamine ↑↑ / Glutamate ↑ / GABA ↓	Explosive energy, impulsivity
Hypomania	Dopamine ↑ / GABA ↓ mild	Creativity, productivity
Depression	Serotonin ↓ / Noradrenaline ↓ / GABA ↑	Slowness, hopelessness
Mixed	Dopamine ↑ + Serotonin ↓ + Glutamate ↑	Chaotic energy, suicidal risk

Clinical advantage:

DNP-21-B does not replace scales, it explains them. It allows pharmacological treatment to be adapted to the individual neurochemical pattern.

18.7 Practical Integration

Table 9 presents the main clinical tools used in the evaluation and monitoring of bipolar disorder, integrating traditional quantitative measures with a qualitative interpretation based on the neurochemical profile proposed by the DNP-21-B model, which allows a more precise and personalized approach to diagnosis and treatment.

Table 9. Clinical instruments for the evaluation of bipolar disorder and its neurochemical correlate (DNP-21-B model)

Tool	Evaluate	Quantitative value	Qualitative value (DNP-21-B)
YMRS	Mania	Intensity of symptoms	Hyperdopaminergia/ hypogaba
MDQ	Bipolar spectrum	Episode history	Dopamine-serotonin oscillation
HCL-32	Hypomania	Functional level	Mild dopaminergic potentiation
CGI-BP	Therapeutic progress	Clinician Insight	Global Neurochemical Balance
DNP-21-B	Biobasis	Neurotransmitter map	Pharmacological personalization

The interview listens to the story. Scales measure the present. DNP-21-B reveals the invisible root (Figure 17).

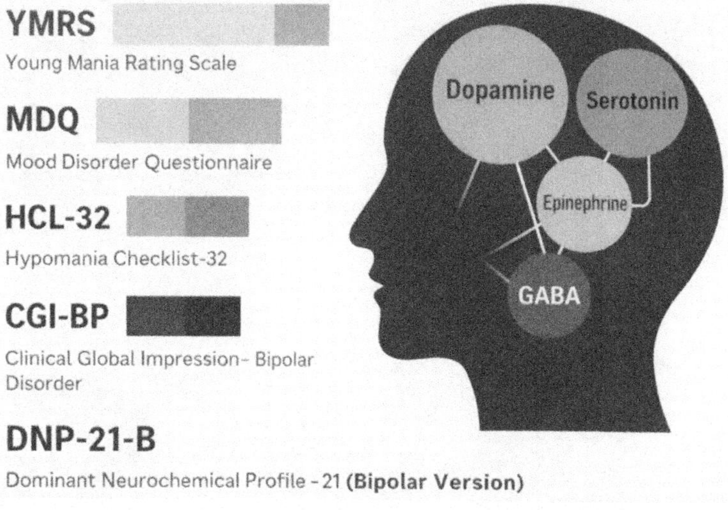

Figure 17. The image symbolizes the integration between clinical assessment and neurochemical understanding: the harmony between measurement and meaning.

18.8 Science that Listens

The scales are the instruments; the DNP-21-B is the score. Only when both are performed together does the true diagnostic melody emerge. Science measures, psychiatry understands, and DNP-21-B translates the chemical soul of the mind.

CHAPTER 19
Differential Diagnosis: ADHD, Borderline, Schizophrenia and Unipolar Depression

Learn to distinguish fire from brightness, and sadness from fall.

19.1 Bipolarity in Disguise

Bipolar disorder does not always present as an obvious cyclone of mania and depression. Sometimes it hides behind symptoms that seem something else: irritability, impulsivity, distractibility or fatigue. For this reason, its differential diagnosis is one of the most delicate tasks of contemporary psychiatry.

Many patients live for years with an incorrect diagnosis, treated for "anxiety" or "depression", until someone asks not only how they feel today, but how they have changed over time.

19.2 Bipolar Disorder versus Unipolar Depression

Both conditions share sadness, hopelessness, and mental slowness, but the key difference is in the history of mood. Table 10 compares bipolar depression and unipolar depression, integrating classic clinical characteristics with the neurochemical profile proposed by the DNP-21-B model, highlighting differences in onset, energy pattern, sleep, family history, and response to SSRIs, fundamental aspects to avoid diagnostic and therapeutic errors.

Table 10. Clinical and Neurochemical Differences Between Bipolar Depression and Unipolar Depression (DNP-21-B Model)

Feature	Bipolar	Unipolar
Onset	Early, episodic	Late, continuous
Energy pattern	Fluctuates: excess and deficit	Always low

Feature	Bipolar	Unipolar
Sleep	Variable	Stable hypersomnia or insomnia
Family History	High bipolar load	More depressive history
Response to SSRIs	Risk of manic swerving	Generally favorable
DNP-21-B Profile	Oscillating dopamine, unstable GABA	Sustained low serotonin

Clinically:

Bipolar people relate times when "everything was easy" or "I felt like I couldn't stop". The unipolar, on the other hand, knows only one emotional tone: gray and constant. In bipolar depression, the soul remembers having flown; in the unipolar, it never took off.

19.3 Bipolar Disorder versus ADHD

ADHD and bipolar share symptoms such as impulsivity, distractibility, and variable energy. However, their rhythms are different: ADHD is constant, bipolarity is cyclical.

Below is a comparison between ADHD and bipolar disorder, two entities that may share symptoms of impulsivity and emotional dysregulation.

Table 11 highlights key differences in onset, clinical course, sleep pattern, emotional expression, response to stimulants, and neurochemical profile according to the DNP-21-B model, which facilitates differential diagnosis and safe therapeutic selection.

Table 11. Clinical and Neurochemical Differences Between ADHD and Bipolar Disorder (DNP-21-B Model)

Appearance	ADHD	Bipolar
Home	Childhood	Adolescence or early adulthood

Appearance	ADHD	Bipolar
Course	Stable, daily	Episodic, with phases
Sleep	Chronic difficulty sleeping	Intermittent insomnia or hypersomnia
Excitement	Reactive, brief	Prolonged, intense
Response to stimulants	Improves concentration	Can induce mania
DNP-21-B	Low Dopamine + Low Noradrenaline	Dopaminafluctuante + Glutamato variable

Example:

A 25 years old man diagnosed with ADHD reports weeks of euphoria alternating with deep sadness. DNP-21-B shows dopaminergic oscillations, confirming type II bipolar with symptoms of secondary inattention.

19.4 Bipolar Disorder versus Borderline Personality Disorder

Borderline and bipolarity are confused by their emotional instability, but their origin is different. In the bipolar, the oscillation is born from neurochemical circuits; in the borderline, from early affective wounds.

Table 12 compares bipolar disorder and borderline personality disorder, two conditions frequently confused in clinical practice. Differences: in the duration of mood swings, identity stability, relational pattern, impulsivity, and neurochemical profile according to the DNP-21-B model are highlighted, which is essential for an accurate differential diagnosis and an appropriate therapeutic approach.

Table 12. Clinical and Neurochemical Differences between Bipolar Disorder and Borderline Personality Disorder (DNP-21-B Model)

Feature	Bipolar	Borderline
Duration of mood swings	Days or weeks	Hours or minutes

Feature	Bipolar	Borderline
Identity	Stable between episodes	Fragmented, changing
Relationships	Intense but stable	Chaotic, afraid of abandonment
Impulsivity	Episodic	Reactive
DNP-21-B	Dopamine-GABA fluctuations	Chronic low serotonin + high cortisol

Example:

A patient diagnosed as borderline shows prolonged phases of euphoria followed by depression and disturbed sleep. The DNP-21-B confirms cyclic dopaminergic alterations → diagnosis adjusted to bipolarity with intense affective traits. The borderline reacts to the bond; the bipolar reacts to the inner rhythm of the brain.

19.5 Bipolar Disorder versus Schizophrenia

Both can include psychotic symptoms, but psychotic bipolarity maintains an emotional connection to reality. The content of the delirium is congruent with the mood.

The following is a comparison between bipolar disorder with psychotic symptoms and schizophrenia, two entities that may have similar psychotic manifestations. Table 13 highlights the differences in the pattern of onset, delusional content, affectivity, functional recovery, and neurochemical profile according to the DNP-21-B model, which allows for accurate diagnostic differentiation and appropriate therapeutic management.

Table 13. Clinical and Neurochemical Differences between Bipolar Disorder with Psychosis and Schizophrenia (DNP-21-B Model)

Feature	Bipolar with psychosis	Schizophrenia
Onset	Episodic, with affective phases	Progressive, continuous

Feature	Bipolar with psychosis	Schizophrenia
Delusions	Emotionally congruent	Incongruous and absurd
Affectivity	Present, intense	Flattened the absent
Recovery	Complete between episodes	Partial or deteriorating
DNP-21-B	Episodic high dopamine	Chronic high dopamine + Dysfunctional Glutamate

Example:

A patient who, during mania, feels "talking to God", and after stabilizing recovers criticism, suffers from bipolar with congruent psychosis. The schizophrenic, on the other hand, keeps the delusional ideas beyond the mood.

19.6 Other Common Confusions

- Generalized anxiety disorder: The mental acceleration of bipolar may seem like anxiety, but in it worry is mixed with euphoria or extreme fatigue.
- Substance abuse disorder: Many times the drug does not cause the disorder, but the bipolar patient seeks to regulate his mood.
- Cyclothymia versus temperament: Cyclothymia is a mild subtype of the bipolar spectrum, with chronic ups and downs without severe functional loss.

19.7 The DNP-21-B as a Differentiation Tool

DNP-21-B provides an objective map of dominant neurotransmitters, allowing for the distinction of conditions similar in presentation, but distinct in their root.

Table 14 integrates different psychiatric disorders from a functional neurochemical perspective, identifying the dominant neurotransmitter, the underlying DNP-21-B pattern, and the main therapeutic orientation, which offers a clinical framework for the personalization of treatment beyond the categorical diagnosis.

Table 14. Psychiatric disorders, neurochemical dominance and therapeutic orientation according to the DNP-21-B model

Disorder	Dominant neurotransmitter	Pattern DNP-21-B	Therapeutic Guidance
Bipolarity	Oscillating dopamine	Dopamine-GABA fluctuation	Dopaminergic stabilization
ADHD	Low noradrenaline	Dopamine-noradrenaline deficiency	Controlled stimulation
Borderline	Low serotonin + high cortisol	Neuroendocrine stress	Emotional psychotherapy + SSRIs
Schizophrenia	High glutamate + chronic dopamine	Limbic-cortical disconnection	Antipsychotic + neuroprotection
Unipolar depression	Stable low serotonin	Pure serotonergic deficit	ISRS + integrative psychotherapy

In this way, DNP-21-B allows pharmacotherapy to be personalized and diagnostic errors to be reduced.

19.8 Diagnose with Accuracy and Compassion

The differential diagnosis of bipolar disorder is not a war of labels, but a search for biographical and neurochemical truth. Each patient is a different symphony: some sound faster, others slower, but all seek tuning.

To distinguish is not to divide: it is to understand. And to understand the bipolar patient is to recognize that behind the fire or shadow, there is always an attempt by the brain to rediscover its natural rhythm (Figure 18).

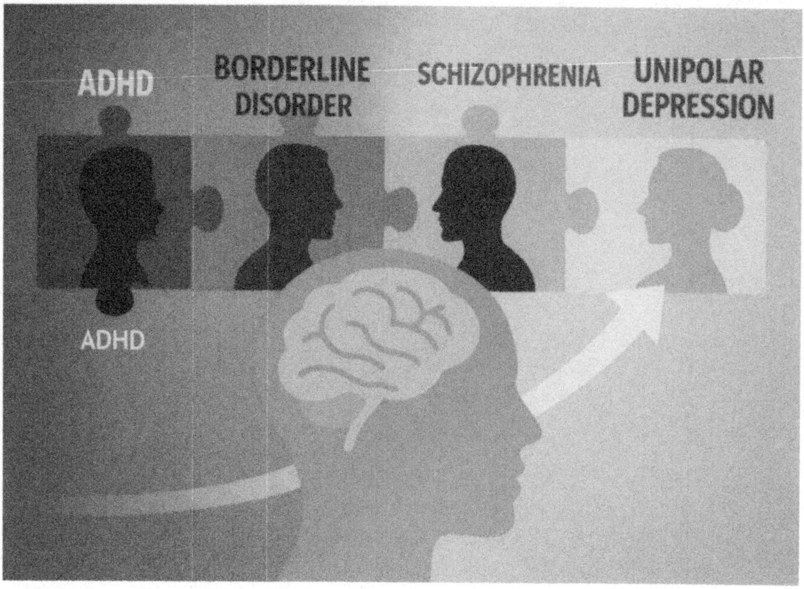

Figure 18. Conceptual representation of the differential diagnosis of bipolar disorder. The image symbolizes the complexity of distinguishing between ADHD, borderline, schizophrenia, and unipolar depression. It shows how clinical and neurochemical boundaries can overlap and become confused.

CHAPTER 20
Bipolar Disorder in Children, Adolescents and Older Adults

Bipolarity through human development:
from youthful fire to cerebral twilight.

20.1 Same Storm, Different Ages

Bipolar disorder does not have a single form or a single time. It can ignite in childhood like a bolt of overflowing energy, manifest itself in adolescence with extreme passions or be reactivated in old age with nuances of irritability, confusion or apathy.

Bipolarity is not a diagnosis, but a vital rhythm that is expressed differently depending on the stage of brain development. Modern neurobiological research has shown that prefrontal cortex maturation, synaptic plasticity, dopaminergic regulation, and neuroinflammation vary with age, modifying clinical presentation and therapeutic response.

20.2 Bipolar Disorder in Childhood. The Energy that the Brain cannot yet Tame

During childhood, the brain is in full synaptic expansion. The dopamine and glutamate systems are not yet balanced, while the limbic (emotional) circuit matures earlier than the prefrontal (rational) cortex. Therefore, emotional regulation depends more on intensity than on reflection.

Common clinical features:

- Chronic irritability or outbursts of anger with no apparent cause.
- Episodes of brief euphoria: excessive laughter, verbiage, minimal need for sleep.
- Multiple mood swings in the same day.
- Risky or aggressive behaviors for their age.
- High creativity, emotional sensitivity, and magical thinking.

Essential differential:

It must be distinguished from ADHD, oppositional defiant disorder and autism spectrum disorders.

Children's DNP-21-B:

- Dopamine ↑, GABA ↓, unstable serotonin.
- Excitatory predominance with poor cortical inhibition.

Intervention:

- Family psychotherapy and psychoeducation.
- Mood stabilizers in moderate-severe cases (valproate, lamotrigine).
- Avoid stimulants without prior neurochemical evaluation.

The bipolar child is not a spoiled child: it is a hyperconnected brain trying to learn to self-regulate its inner fire.

20.3 Bipolar Disorder in Adolescence. The Brain in Metamorphosis

In adolescence, dopamine reaches its physiological peak, which increases novelty-seeking, risk, and impulsivity. The maturation of the frontal lobe has not yet completed its inhibitory function, leading to an imbalance between emotion and control.

Characteristic symptoms:

- Alternation between expansive euphoria and despair.
- Self-destructive behaviors, alcohol or cannabis abuse.
- Feeling "invincible" or "not needing sleep".
- Existential and creative crises of great intensity.

Neurobiology:

- High dopaminergic and glutamatergic tone.
- Transient decrease in GABA and serotonin.
- High vulnerability to psychosocial stress (hyperreactive orbitofrontal cortex).

Clinical example:

A 16 years old boy, once an excellent student, begins to write at night, does not sleep, speaks quickly and plans multiple ventures. DNP-21-B confirms dopamine ↑↑, GABA ↓: classic hypomanic phase.

Treatment:

- Emotional education, family therapy and sleep routine.
- Lithium as a reference stabilizer.
- Academic and digital supervision (avoid overexposure to screens and networks).

In bipolar adolescence, art can be a refuge or catharsis. The clinician's task is to transform chaos into creativity.

20.4 Bipolar Disorder in Adulthood. The Possible Balance

In adulthood, the brain reaches its greatest integration between emotion and cognition.

However, bipolar episodes can affect the structure and function of the white matter, especially in the corpus callosum and anterior cingulate, interfering with the connection between hemispheres.

Clinical manifestations:

- Clearly delimited phases of mania, hypomania or depression.
- Functional impact on work and family.
- Increased awareness of the disorder and desire for stability.

DNP-21-B in adult:

- More defined dopamine–GABA cycles.
- Serotonergic predominance in recovery.
- Optimal response to mood stabilizers + mind-body therapies.

Intervention:

- Cognitive-behavioral psychotherapy adapted to the bipolar spectrum.
- Regular monitoring of EKG, plasma levels, and sleep.
- Aerobic physical activity and mindfulness as natural dopaminergic modulators.

20.5 Bipolar Disorder in the Elderly. The Storm under the Calm

The aging brain experiences loss of synaptic plasticity, decreased dopamine and serotonin, and increased oxidative stress and neuroinflammation. This modifies the expression of bipolar disorder, making it more attenuated, but more resistant to treatment.

Common symptoms:

- Prolonged depressive episodes and low response to antidepressants.
- "Silent" manias (fast talking, irritability, compulsive shopping).
- Cognitive alterations or affective pseudodementia.
- Increased cardiovascular risk and drug interactions.

DNP-21-B geriatric acid:

- Dopamine ↓↓, serotonin ↓, GABA ↑, glutamate ↑.
- Neurochemical profile of inflammation and mitochondrial energy reduction.

Treatment:

- Low doses of atypical stabilizers and antipsychotics.
- Adapted physical exercise and cognitive stimulation.
- Anti-inflammatory diet (omega-3, turmeric, red fruits).

In bipolar old age, energy no longer burns: it flickers, but it can still illuminate if it is cared for with scientific tenderness.

20.6 Neuroevolutionary Approach. The Dopamine Cycle and Emotional Wisdom

Throughout life, bipolarity follows a neuroevolutionary curve:

- Childhood: overflowing dopamine without cortical brake.
- Adolescence: dopamine and glutamate in creative expansion.
- Adulthood: dopamine and GABA in dynamic balance.
- Old age: dopamine in decline, GABA in excess, fragile serotonin.

The clinical challenge is to adapt the treatment to the patient's neurobiological moment. The DNP-21-B makes it possible to observe how brain chemistry changes with age and adjust medication with pinpoint precision.

20.7 The Same Melody in Different Keys

Bipolar disorder does not belong to an age; it belongs to the human being. Its expression varies like a melody that is repeated throughout life, but in different tones and speeds.

In childhood, the brain learns to feel. In adolescence, to explore. In adulthood, to be sustained. In old age, to understand. Each stage has its own challenge, and modern psychiatry —armed with science, empathy, and neurochemistry— has a duty to accompany that journey with respect, precision, and hope (Figure 19).

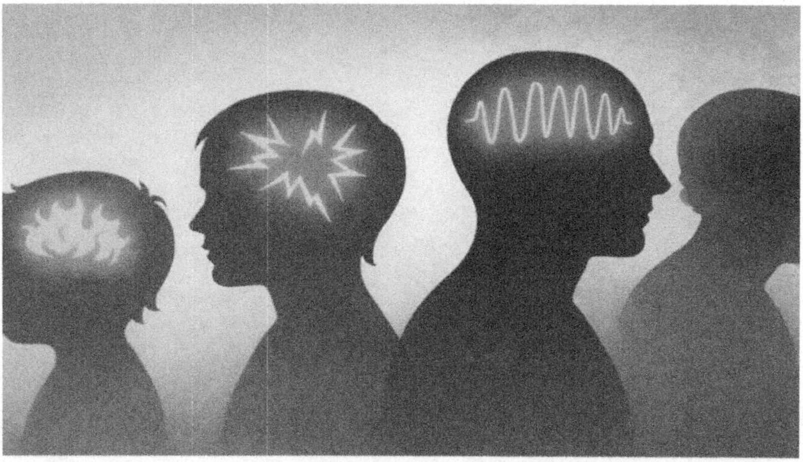

Figure 19. Conceptual representation of bipolar disorder throughout the life cycle. The image shows how his expression changes from the overflowing energy of childhood, through the emotional storm of adolescence to the balance of adulthood and the serenity of old age.

CHAPTER 21
Most Common Errors in Diagnosing Bipolar Disorder

When haste extinguishes clinical truth.

21.1 The Cost of Late Diagnosis

Recent studies estimate that it takes between 7 and 10 years for a patient with bipolar disorder to receive a correct diagnosis. During that time, most are treated as “depressed”, “anxious”, or “emotionally unstable”.

The cost of that delay is not only clinical: it is existential. Each misdiagnosis robs years of stability and sows distrust in medicine. Understanding the most frequent mistakes does not seek to point out culprits, but to recover empathic precision, where science and listening are reconciled.

21.2 Mistake 1: Confusing Bipolar with Unipolar Depression

The most common mistake is to diagnose depression without exploring the manic or hypomanic past. The clinician asks, “Are you sad?” but forgets to ask, “Have you had times when you felt too good?”.

Consequences:

- Treatment with antidepressants that can induce mania.
- Faster oscillations (fast cycles).
- The patient's feeling of “getting better and then getting worse for no reason”.

Example:

A 32 years old woman treated for 5 years for major depression enters the manic phase after SSRIs. DNP-21-B re-evaluation → dopamine ↑↑, GABA ↓ → diagnosis adjusted to type II bipolarity. Bipolar depression is recognized when one looks not only for sadness, but for the history of the fire that preceded it.

21.3 Mistake 2: Labeling as ADHD what is Juvenile Bipolar

ADHD is a fashionable diagnosis, but juvenile bipolar often mimics your hyperactivity, impulsivity, and distractibility. The difference is in the cyclicality and deep emotionality.

Differentiating keys:

- ADHD is constant; the bipolar, fluctuating.
- Bipolar can go from hyperactivity to crying for no apparent reason.
- Stimulants aggravate bipolar symptoms.

DNP-21-B:

- ADHD → low dopamine and low norepinephrine.
- Bipolarity → oscillating dopamine and high glutamate.

Consequence of the error:

Medicating a bipolar child with stimulants can precipitate mania or extreme irritability.

21.4 Mistake 3: Confusing with Borderline Personality Disorder

The borderline has emotional reactivity to bonds; the bipolar, neurochemical internal rhythms. Both can coexist, but confusion arises when the oscillation is interpreted as a psychological drama rather than a biological phenomenon.

Example:

A patient with intense emotional changes, diagnosed with borderline, but with episodes of three weeks without sleep and accelerated speech. DNP-21-B confirms hyperdopaminergia → bipolarity. The limit is not in the personality, but in the synapse.

21.5 Mistake 4: Ignoring the Biological and Neurochemical Component

Many diagnoses are made only from the verbal interview, without integrating laboratory tests, EKG or DNP-21-B profile. Modern psychiatry demands looking at the biology of emotion.

Common mistakes:

- Attributing everything to "childhood traumas".
- Not evaluating sleep, thyroid, inflammation, or circadian rhythm.
- Discard the role of lithium or stabilizers due to prejudice.

Example:

Patient with an unstable mood, very low vitamin D and high dopamine → after metabolic correction, the episodes decrease. Not all emotional instability is psychological; many times it is bioelectric.

21.6 Mistake 5: Diagnosing Generalized Anxiety Instead of Hypomania

Hypomania is often confused with anxiety because both states share mental acceleration and lack of sleep. But the difference lies in the emotional valence:

- In anxiety there is fear.
- In hypomania there is pleasure, urgency and creativity.

Clinical example:

A lawyer sleeps four hours, works without a break, and feels "her mind enlightened". The initial diagnosis was anxiety, but DNP-21-B shows elevated dopamine and glutamate → hypomania.

21.7 Mistake 6: Believing that the Patient Exaggerates or Manipulates

Nothing damages the therapeutic alliance more than prejudice. The bipolar patient may seem inconsistent, but it is actually consistent with his or her neurochemical state at the time.

Minimizing their narrative is equivalent to losing an opportunity for prevention. What the clinician calls "drama" may actually be a synaptic storm.

21.8 Mistake 7: Not Educating the Patient or Family

The diagnosis does not end when it is written in the file. The real work begins when the patient understands their disease and participates in its treatment. Without education, adherence falls, and the cycle begins again.

Keys:

- Explain that bipolarity is biological and treatable.
- Teach how to identify early signs of relapse.
- Involve the family without guilt or stigma.

21.9 DNP-21-B as an Antidote to Diagnostic Error

The dominant neurochemical profile (DNP-21-B) helps to:

- Differentiate bipolar from other affective pathologies.
- Predict response to stabilizing drugs.
- Avoid counterproductive treatments.
- Identify neurochemical subtypes (dopaminergic, serotonergic, glutamatergic).

Example:

A patient with a doubtful diagnosis between ADHD and type II bipolar. DNP-21-B shows high dopamine, low GABA, → confirms bipolar dopaminergic pattern. DNP-21-B not only helps diagnose, but also restores trust between doctor and patient (Figure 20).

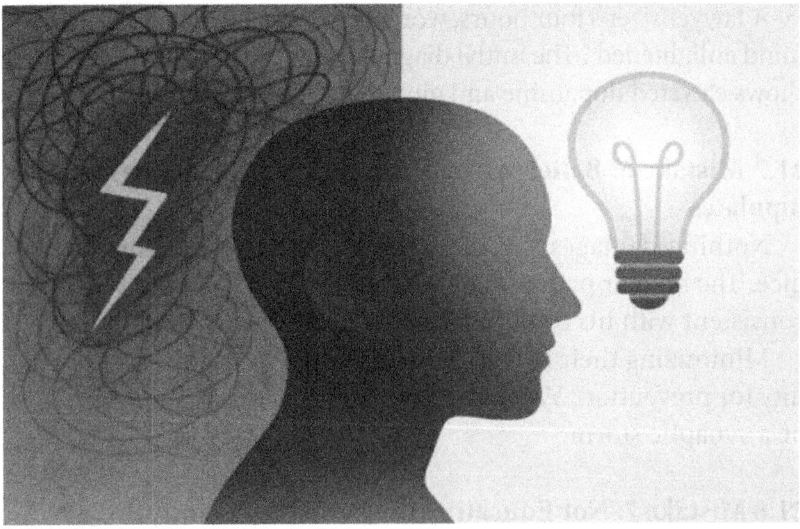

Figure 20. Conceptual representation of diagnostic errors in bipolar disorder. The image symbolizes the shift from confusion and stigma to clinical clarity, showing how scientific understanding and empathy illuminate what was previously misunderstood.

21.10 Diagnose with Humility and Depth

Diagnosing well is an act of humility. It means admitting that the human mind does not fit into fixed categories, but into complex biological rhythms. The diagnostic error is sometimes unavoidable, but it can be corrected when the clinician decides to listen not only to the patient, but also to the biology that inhabits him. The correct diagnosis is not only a clinical act: it is an act of justice towards the suffering mind.

PART V.
Pharmacological Treatment

CHAPTER 22
Mood Stabilizers: Lithium, Valproate, Lamotrigine and Carbamazepine

The pillars of neurochemical balance.

22.1 The Chemistry of Stability

If antidepressants are the drugs of emotion, mood stabilizers are the drugs of rhythm. They do not seek to elevate or extinguish, but to restore the natural frequency of the mood. Its purpose is not to flatten emotion, but to make it habitable. A good stabilizer is not a chemical prison, but an anchor that allows the soul to sail without being shipwrecked.

Among all the available treatments, lithium, valproate, lamotrigine and carbamazepine remain the four classic pillars of bipolar therapy. Each one represents a different mechanism within the orchestra of neurotransmission acting not only on symptoms, but on the biological architecture of emotional regulation.

22.2 Lithium, the Element of Balance

Discovered in the mid-20th century, lithium remains one of the oldest and most effective treatments in psychiatry. A simple mineral ion that modulates neuronal excitability by stabilizing sodium and calcium channels.

Mechanisms of action:

- It regulates intracellular signaling by inhibiting GSK-3β.
- BDNF (brain neurotrophic factor) increases.
- Restores circadian gene expression.
- Reduces dopaminergic hyperactivity and glutamate toxicity.

Clinical indications:

- Bipolar disorder type I (mania, mixed, maintenance).
- Suicide prevention (the only drug with this effect proven).
- Enhancer in resistant depressions.

DNP-21-B correlation:

- Decreases dopaminergic peaks.
- Increases GABAergic tone.
- Promotes neuroplastic homeostasis.

Monitoring:

- Plasma levels: 0.6–1.2 mEq/L (maintenance).
- Periodic monitoring of renal function, thyroid and EKG.
- Hydration and Sodium Balance Essential for Safety.

Side effects:

Fine tremor, mild thirst, hypothyroidism, kidney sensitivity. Lithium is not just a drug: it is the mineral heartbeat of psychiatry, the bridge between emotion and chemistry.

22.3 Valproate. The Shield of Inhibition

Valproic acid acts mainly by enhancing GABAergic inhibition and reducing neuronal hyperexcitability. It is especially useful in patients with rapid cycles or mixed episodes, where dopamine and glutamate are overactive.

Mechanisms:

- Inhibits the degradation of GABA.
- Blocks voltage-gated sodium channels.
- It epigenetically modulates gene expression (histone deacetylase inhibition).

Clinical Uses:

- Acute mania and maintenance.
- Mixed states and severe irritability.
- Comorbidity with addictions or impulsivity.

DNP-21-B correlation:

- Reinforces GABA.
- Decreases glutamate and dopamine.
- Regulates limbic hyperreactivity.

Side effects:

Weight gain, hair loss, mild tremor, liver alteration (requires enzyme control).

Valproate represents the calm after the storm: the neurochemical brake that prevents emotion from burning its own circuit.

22.4 Lamotrigine. The Light and Shadow Stabilizer

Lamotrigine does not sedate or accelerate: it regulates transitions. Its greatest effectiveness lies in preventing depressive phases, which is why it is recommended in type II bipolar and predominantly depressive cycles.

Mechanisms:

- Inhibits voltage-gated sodium channels.
- Reduces glutamate release.
- Promotes cortical synchrony.

Clinical profile:

- Prevention of depressive phases.
- Excellent tolerance, no weight gain.
- Limited effectiveness for mania.

DNP-21-B correlation:

- Decreases glutamatergic overexcitation.
- Balances serotonin and glutamate.
- Reinforces cortical stability.

Precautions:

Slow titration to avoid skin rash (rare Stevens-Johnson syndrome). Lamotrigine acts as a conductor between emotional extremes: it restores rhythm without shutting down melody.

22.5 Carbamazepine. The Guardian of Neuronal Fire

Initially developed as an anticonvulsant, carbamazepine stabilizes neuronal firing by modulating sodium channels and reducing glutamate. It is useful in mixed or dysphoric episodes, especially in patients who cannot tolerate lithium or valproate.

Mechanisms:

- Reduces sodium-dependent depolarization.
- Increases the release of serotonin.
- It inhibits limbic hyperexcitability.

DNP-21-B correlation:

- Decreases glutamate.
- Stabilizes noradrenergic tone.
- Restores balance in chaotic oscillations.

Side effects:

Drowsiness, dizziness, mild ataxia, rare agranulocytosis (periodic blood count check). Carbamazepine is the silent guardian: less famous than lithium, but often the one who restores peace to restless neurons.

22.6 Choosing the Right Stabilizer

Each brain dances with its own neurochemical rhythm. Choosing a stabilizer requires understanding not only the diagnosis, but the dominant neurotransmitter profile revealed by DNP-21-B.

Table 15 relates the predominant neurochemical profiles to the most appropriate mood stabilizer and its main therapeutic action, which offers a clinical guideline aimed at the personalization of pharmacological treatment in bipolar disorder according to the DNP-21-B model.

Table 15. Selection of mood stabilizers according to neurochemical profile (model DNP-21-B)

Neurochemical profile	Ideal stabilizer	Main Action
Dopaminergic dominance	Lithium	Antimanic, reduces impulse

Neurochemical profile	Ideal stabilizer	Main Action
Glutamatergic dominance	Lamotrigine o Carbamazepine	Antidepressant, neuroprotective
GABAergic deficiency	Valproate	Antiimpulsive, calming
Serotonergic deficit	Lamotrigine	Mood regulator
Mixed (high dopamine + glutamate)	Combination (Lithium + Valproate)	Dual modulation

DNP-21-B allows for precision psychiatry, where treatment aligns with the brain's internal symphony rather than fighting it.

22.7 Integrative and Future Perspectives

Research shows that stabilizers not only control symptoms, but protect the brain structurally. Neuroimaging studies (MRI, PET) reveal increased gray matter volume and increased synaptic resilience in patients treated long-term with lithium and lamotrigine.

Pop-up addresses:

- Biomarker-guided dosing (BDNF, cytokines).
- Neuroinflammatory modulation (microglia and cytokines).
- Combined therapies with nutraceuticals (omega-3, N-acetylcysteine, turmeric).

The goal of modern psychiatry is not only to prevent relapse, but to cultivate neuroresilience: a brain capable of learning to repair itself.

22.8 The Science of Balance

Mood stabilizers remind us that emotion is not the enemy of reason, but its companion. These molecules —born from chemistry and perfected by clinical experience—constitute the scaffolding on which millions of people rebuild their stability. Treating bipolarity is not about suppressing emotion, but about teaching it to breathe harmoniously (Figure 21).

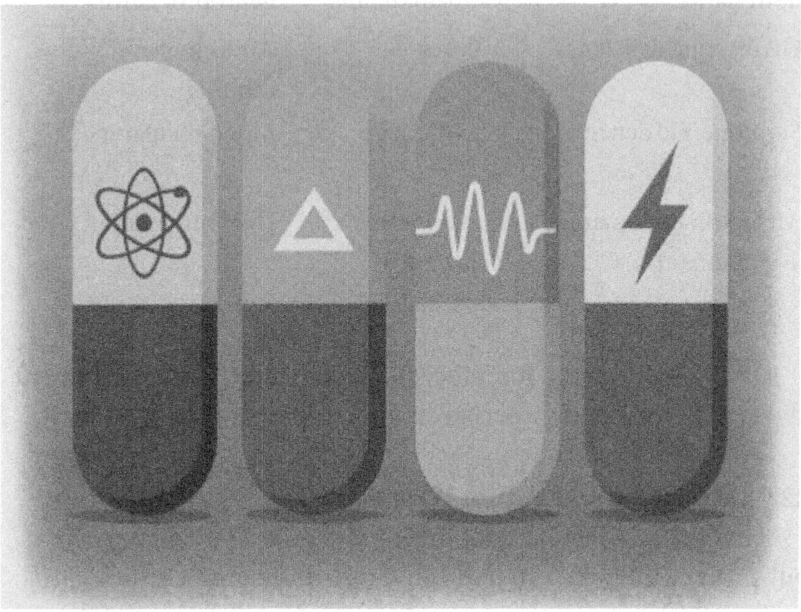

Figure 21. Conceptual representation of mood stabilizers: lithium, valproate, lamotrigine and carbamazepine. The image symbolizes the neurochemical harmony achieved when the brain manages to regulate its own cycles of energy and calm.

CHAPTER 23
Atypical Antipsychotics: Quetiapine, Olanzapine, Lurasidone and Aripiprazole

Between dopamine and serenity: the modulators of the bipolar soul.

23.1 When Excess Dopamine Turns to Noise

Bipolarity is a chemical dance between excitement and containment. In the manic phases, dopamine rises like an overflowing river; thoughts speed up, judgment scatters, and sleep evaporates. This is where atypical antipsychotics are born, drugs that do not "turn off" the mind, butre-establish the filter between thought and reality.

The modern antipsychotic does not seek to silence the mind, but to restore the ability to hear clearly. These drugs work primarily by modulating dopamine (D2) and serotonin (5-HT2A) receptors, creating a pharmacological symphony that reduces overstimulation without destroying creativity.

23.2 Quetiapine: the Inner Storm Soothing

Quetiapine is perhaps the most versatile antipsychotic on the bipolar spectrum. Its action extends from acute mania to bipolar depression, thanks to its balance between dopaminergic antagonism and serotonergic action.

Main mechanisms:

- It blocks D2 and 5-HT_2A receptors → reduces dopamine and relieves mania.
- It activates 5-HT_1A receptors → antidepressant and anxiolytic effect.
- Active metabolite (norquetiapine) inhibits norepinephrine reuptake.

Clinical Uses:

- Mania, bipolar depression and maintenance.
- Resistant insomnia and associated anxiety.

Side effects:

- Drowsiness, weight gain, mild hypotension.

DNP-21-B correlation:

- Dopamine ↓ moderate.
- Serotonin ↑
- GABA ↑ → balancing profile in mixed phases.

Quetiapine is like a night's rest after days of euphoria: it restores silence without extinguishing life.

23.3 Olanzapine: the Energy Stabilizer

Olanzapine is a potent atypical antipsychotic with action on dopamine, serotonin, histamine, and acetylcholine. It is ideal for intense manic phases or patients with irritability and behavioral uncontrol.

Mechanisms:

- D2 and 5-HT_2A Block → powerful anti-manic effect.
- It increases dopamine in the prefrontal cortex → improves cognition.
- Reduces cortisol and physiological anxiety.

Applications:

- Acute mania, maintenance.
- Fluoxetine is associated with bipolar depression.

Adverse effects:

- Weight gain, insulin resistance, drowsiness.

DNP-21-B correlation:

- Subcortical dopamine decreases.
- Increases frontal dopamine.
- Balances serotonin and norepinephrine.

Olanzapine represents the power of brain rest: its effect is profound, but it demands metabolic discipline.

23.4 Lurasidone: Clarity without Sedation

Lurasidone belongs to the new generation of antipsychotics with a cleaner profile.

It is one of the few approved for bipolar depression, and its action does not block creativity or cause excessive sleepiness.

Mechanisms:

- Antagonism 5-HT2A and D2.
- 5-HT1A partial agonism (antidepressant and anxiolytic effect).
- Cortical glutamatergic modulation.

Advantages:

- It does not gain weight.
- Improves cognitive functions.
- Safe metabolic profile.

DNP-21-B:

- Dopamine ↓ selective.
- Serotonin ↑ regulated.
- Stabilized glutamate.

Lurassidone is lucid balance: it calms without shutting down, regulates without numbing.

23.5 Aripiprazole: the Dopaminergic System Modulator

Aripiprazole is not a pure antagonist, but a partial agonist: it acts as a "chemical thermostat", reducing dopamine when there is too much and stimulating it when it is lacking.

Mechanisms:

- Partial agonist D2 and 5-HTA.
- 5-HT2A antagonist.
- It normalizes dopamine in all pathways.

Indications:

- Mania, maintenance, relapse prevention.
- Excellent choice for adolescents and overweight patients.

Side effects:

- Restlessness, mild insomnia, occasional impulsivity.

DNP-21-B correlation:

- It regulates dopamine bidirectionally.
- Maintains stable serotonin.
- Reduces frontal hyper-reactivity.

Aripiprazole does not turn off dopamine: it educates it.

23.6 DNP-21-B Selection

Table 16 links the neurochemical profiles defined by the DNP-21-B model with the rational choice of antipsychotic and its main clinical objective, which facilitates a more precise therapeutic approach in the different phases of bipolar disorder and its comorbidities.

Table 16. Selection of antipsychotics according to DNP-21-B neurochemical profile and clinical objective

DNP-21-B Profile	Ideal antipsychotic	Clinical objective
Very high dopamine	Olanzapine or quetiapine	Mania Control
High Dopamine + High Glutamate	Lurasidone	Bipolar depression
Unstable dopamine	Aripiprazol	Cognitive stabilization
Low GABA + Low Serotonin	Quetiapina	Anxiety + insomnia

The use of antipsychotics should be understood not as "chemical blockade", but as tuning of the dopaminergic system. The DNP-21-B guides the choice with neurophysiological precision and prevents both over-sedation and relapse.

23.7 Beyond the Stigma

For decades, the word "antipsychotic" generated fear. But modern science shows that these drugs preserve brain structure, reduce inflammation, and improve neuroplasticity when used judiciously. The true antipsychotic is not the one that erases the mind, but the one that returns it to its axis.

23.8 The Art of Modulating Dopamine

Treatment with atypical antipsychotics requires balance, observation, and empathy. Each molecule has its character: the calmness of quetiapine, the strength of olanzapine, the clarity of lurasidone, and the intelligence of aripiprazole (Figure 22).

All of them, together, allow the bipolar brain to feel again without losing control. Regulating dopamine is like conducting an orchestra: too much intensity confuses, too much stillness saddens. The modern psychiatrist does not silence the symphony, he tunes it.

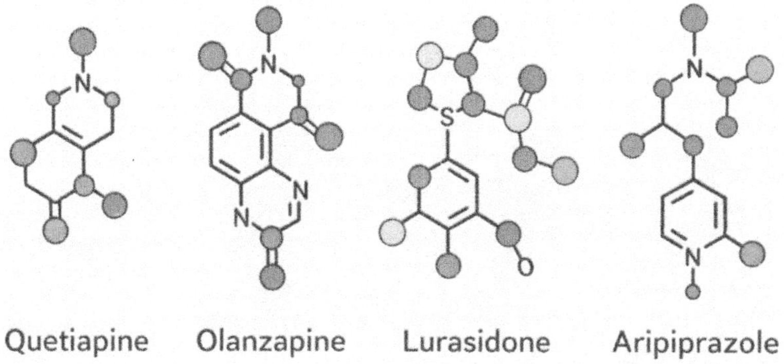

Figure 22. Conceptual representation of the main atypical antipsychotics used in bipolar disorder: quetiapine, olanzapine, lurasidone, and aripiprazole. The image symbolizes the balance between dopamine and serotonin that these drugs help restore.

CHAPTER 24
Cautious Use of Antidepressants in Bipolar Disorder

Between hope and risk:
When lifting your spirits can stir up the storm.

24.1 The Double-Edged Serotonin

Few clinical decisions are as delicate as prescribing an antidepressant to a bipolar patient. In an attempt to relieve hopelessness, the doctor runs the risk of igniting a manic phase.

The balance between relief and relapse thus becomes a form of clinical art, supported by both science and prudence. In bipolar disorder, an antidepressant can be a beacon or a spark. The difference is in the timing, the dose, and the accompaniment.

24.2 Neurochemical Basis: Serotonin, Dopamine, and the Oscillation Axis

The bipolar brain oscillates between excess and deficit. In depression, dopaminergic and serotonergic hypoactivity dominates, but the attempt to correct it with an antidepressant can disrupt the dopamine-GABA balance, triggering mania.

Paradoxical effect:

- Sudden increase in serotonin → inhibits GABA → disinhibits dopamine → hypomania or mania.
- Especially common with SSRIs (fluoxetine, sertraline) or SNRIs (venlafaxine, duloxetine).

DNP-21-B correlation:

- Patient with unstable dopamine or low GABA = high risk of manic turn.
- Patient with pure serotonergic profile = safer use of antidepressants.

The antidepressant should not be given by protocol, but after reading the patient's neurochemical map.

24.3 Types of Antidepressants and Risk of Swerving

Table 17 summarizes the main classes of antidepressants, representative examples, and their relative risk of inducing mania in patients with bipolar disorder. In addition, practical clinical comments are incorporated to guide safe and rational use within a stabilizing therapeutic scheme.

Table 17. Antidepressants and risk of manic turn in the disorder bipolar

Pharmacological class	Examples	Riskof mania	Clinical Comments
SSRIs	Fluoxetine, sertraline, escitalopram	High	Avoid in mixed phase or type I
IRSN	Venlafaxine, duloxetine	Very high	Empower dopamine in directly
Tricyclics	Amitriptyline, imipramine	Very high	Not recommended in bipolarity
MAOOS	Selegilina, tranilcipromina	High	Hypertensive risk and Swerve
Bupropion	Bupropion	Moderate–low	Better tolerance, can be used in type II
Mirtazapine	Mirtazapine	Low	Safe with stabilize-concomitant

No antidepressant is innocent: its safety depends on the neurochemical context and the protection of the stabilizer.

24.4 The Golden Rule: Never in Monotherapy

The most frequent and dangerous mistake is to prescribe an antidepressant without a mood stabilizer. Clinical evidence shows that this practice doubles the risk of rapid cycling and mania.

Clinical principle:

- All antidepressants must be accompanied by lithium, valproate or lamotrigine.
- In mild bipolar depression, it is recommended to prioritize psychotherapy and melatonin before resorting to medication.

Clinical example:

A patient with bipolar depression type II treated with sertraline without stabilizer presents insomnia, irritability and verbiage. SSRI was discontinued, lamotrigine was started → stability in 6 weeks. No single molecule can control a brain that lives in oscillation.

24.5 Early Signs of Manic Turning

- Less need for sleep.
- Increased energy or libido.
- Acceleration of thought.
- Rapid speech, euphoria, or irritability.
- Impulsivity or excessive purchases.

Early recognition makes it possible to stop the turn before it consolidates. The physician should educate the patient and family to report sudden changes in energy or sleep.

Predictive DNP-21-B:

A dopamine that rises more than 25% from baseline after 10 days of antidepressant predicts imminent turnaround.

24.6 Strategies for the Prudent Use of Antidepressants

1. Confirm bipolar diagnosis (avoid false unipolar depressions).
2. Evaluate DNP-21-B prior to initiation: if dopamine or glutamate are high, postpone treatment.
3. Start with low doses and slow titration.
4. Always combine with stabilizer.
5. Avoid during mixed phases or recent hypomania.
6. Monitor sleep, energy, impulsivity, and social pressure.

Recommended duration:

- 8 to 12 weeks maximum, with progressive withdrawal.
- Reassess neurochemical profile before restarting.

Bipolar depression does not heal quickly. He paces himself patiently.

24.7 Non-Antidepressant Alternatives for the Bipolar Depressive Phase

- Lamotrigine: best stabilizing option with antidepressant effect.
- Quetiapine or lurasidone: proven efficacy without risk of reversal.
- Biological therapies: TMS, ECT, ketamine (under protocol).
- Interpersonal Therapy and Social Rhythm (IPSRT): Stabilizes sleep and energy.
- Omega-3 and N-acetylcysteine: modulate inflammation and glutamate.

The ideal treatment for the depressed bipolar is not the one that lifts the mood, but the one that returns the rhythm.

24.8 Special Considerations

In pregnancy:

- Avoid high-risk SSRIs (paroxetine). Prefer psychotherapy and lamotrigine.

In the elderly:

- Slow metabolism, increased risk of confusion and side effects.

In adolescents:

- Avoid monotherapy, the turn is more abrupt and emotionally dangerous.

With a history of addiction:

- Avoid stimulant antidepressants (bupropion, venlafaxine).

24.9 Pharmacological Humility

The bipolar antidepressant is a useful tool, but only when used with humility. It is not a matter of fighting sadness at all costs, but of protecting the integrity of the emotional rhythm.

Each bipolar brain has a different balance point, and the psychiatrist's duty is to listen to it before medicating it. In the art of treating bipolar depression, prudence is the highest form of clinical intelligence (Figure 23).

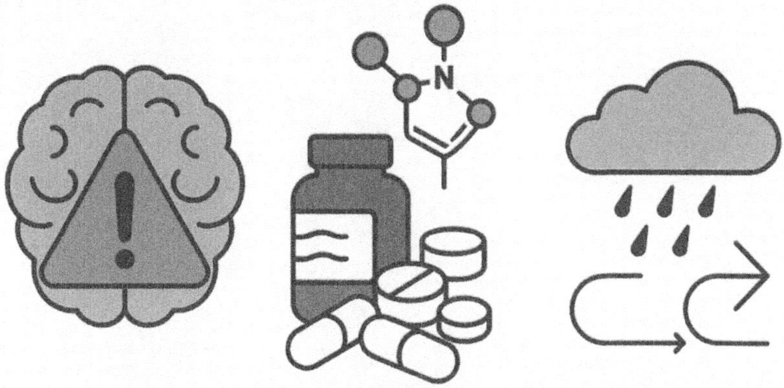

Figure 23. Conceptual representation of the cautious use of antidepressants in bipolar disorder. The image symbolizes the delicate balance between relieving depression and avoiding manic turn, reflecting the fine line between stability and neurochemical dysregulation.

CHAPTER 25
Benzodiazepines, Melatonin and Insomnia Management Associated with Bipolar Disorder

The art of sleeping without shutting down the mind.

25.1 Sleep as a Natural Mood Stabilizer

In the bipolar brain, sleep is not a luxury: it is medicine. Each night represents an opportunity to restore the synchrony between dopamine, serotonin, GABA and melatonin.

When sleep is disturbed, the emotional balance is broken, and the mind, deprived of rest, can enter euphoria or depression. Sleeping well is not escaping from the world, but returning to the biological order that sustains the mind.

Bipolar insomnia does not always come from anxiety or depression: it is often an early marker of turnaround. Therefore, managing it properly is as important a therapeutic intervention as lithium or psychotherapy.

25.2 Neurobiology of Sleep and Bipolarity

Sleep is a coordinated neurochemical rhythm. During deep sleep (N3 phase), GABA inhibits the prefrontal cortex, while melatonin regulates body temperature and dopamine drops to its basal level. In the REM phase, dopamine rises again, facilitating the emotional consolidation of memories.

In the bipolar brain:

- The GABA–glutamate axis is unstable.
- The circadian clock loses synchrony.
- Melatonin secretion is delayed or interrupted.

Result: insomnia, early awakenings or inverted cycles (nocturnal activity and daytime sleepiness). When melatonin is turned off, the soul loses its circadian compass.

25.3 Benzodiazepines. The Nervous System's Brief Respite

Benzodiazepines act on GABA-A receptors, which increases neuronal inhibition. They are useful in phases of acute insomnia, intense anxiety or initial mania.

Clinical examples:

- Lorazepam: intermediate action, ideal for anxiety attacks and restful sleep.
- Clonazepam: long-acting, useful for stabilizing the nighttime rhythm.
- Alprazolam: restricted use, risk of dependence if maintained for more than 4 weeks.

Advantages:

- They induce rapid sleep.
- They calm dopaminergic hyperactivation.

Risks:

- Tolerance, dependence, and residual sleepiness.
- Interference with memory and coordination.

DNP-21-B correlation:

They increase GABA and reduce dopamine, which helps stop phases of early activation, but can decrease motivation if abused. Benzodiazepine does not cure insomnia, it lends it. Its power is in punctual use, not in custom.

25.4 Melatonin. The Molecular Clock of Mood

Melatonin doesn't just regulate sleep; it regulates emotional stability. Its secretion depends on darkness, body temperature, and the signal from the suprachiasmatic nucleus of the hypothalamus.

Key Features:

- Synchronizes the circadian rhythm.
- Regulates dopamine, serotonin, and cortisol.
- Decreases neuroglial inflammation.

Clinical use in bipolarity:

- Dose of 1–3 mg in the evening.
- Complement in depressive phases with insomnia.
- Useful in night shifts or jet lag trips.

DNP-21-B correlation:

Increases GABA, balances dopamine, and reduces cortisol, creating a nocturnal symphony that promotes neuronal repair. Melatonin doesn't induce sleep: it reminds the brain that it's time to rest.

25.5 Non-Pharmacological Strategies for Bipolar Insomnia

- Sleep hygiene: regular schedule, avoiding screens and caffeine at night.
- Light therapy: morning exposure to natural light to reinforce circadian rhythms.
- Mindfulness and diaphragmatic breathing: reduce adrenaline and facilitate sleep.
- Warm baths and slow music: activate the parasympathetic system.
- Avoid sleeping during the day: stay in sync with sunlight.

It should be noted that there is no pill that compensates for the loss of rest rituals.

25.6 Natural Alternatives and Emerging Therapies

- Magnesium and glycine: relax the nervous system and improve deep sleep.
- Valerian and passionflower: increase GABA, useful in mild nighttime anxiety.
- CBD (cannabidiol): anxiolytic and sleep stabilizing effect in low doses.
- Transcranial magnetic stimulation (TMS): improves cortical rhythm in refractory insomnia.

The medicine of the future will not be just chemistry: it will be rhythmic.

25.7 Insomnia as a Sentinel Symptom

In the bipolar patient, insomnia precedes relapse. You can anticipate both a manic and depressive phase. Recording sleep with apps or smartwatches allows the clinician to detect patterns and adjust treatment before collapse.

Alarm indicators:

- Less than 5 hours of sleep for more than 3 nights.
- Morning euphoria or sudden nighttime activity.
- Decreased appetite and increased creative or grandiose ideas.

Poor sleep isn't always tiredness: sometimes it's the prologue to a neurochemical storm.

25.8 Sleep as a Form of Treatment

Sleep is the first therapy and the last frontier of bipolar stability. Taking care of it is as important as adjusting the lithium or quetiapine dosage. The doctor's task is not only to induce sleep, but torestore the neurochemical choreography that makes it possible. Teaching good sleep is teaching the bipolar brain to reconcile with its own night (Figure 24).

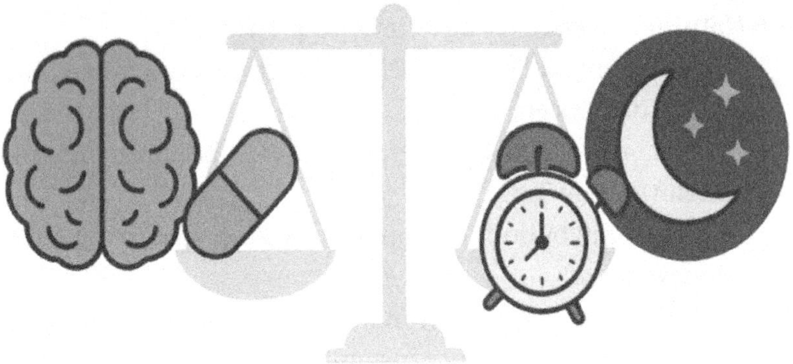

Figure 24. Conceptual representation of the management of insomnia in bipolar disorder. Benzodiazepines and melatonin are shown as elements in a delicate balance, which promotes both rest and caution.

CHAPTER 26
New Biologic Therapies: Ketamine, Esketamine, Psilocybin, ECT and TMS

Neuroplasticity as a new therapeutic horizon.

26.1 From Classical Pharmacology to the Synaptic Revolution

For decades, treatment for bipolar disorder focused on stabilizing mood using lithium, anticonvulsants, or antipsychotics. However, contemporary science has opened a new frontier: the direct stimulation of neuroplasticity, that is, the brain's ability to regenerate synaptic connections and reorganize emotional circuits.

The future of bipolar treatment does not only seek to calm the symptoms, but also to reprogram the neural networks that generate them. These biological therapies—ketamine, esketamine, psilocybin, electroconvulsive therapy (ECT), and transcranial magnetic stimulation (TMS)— are not just alternatives: they represent a neuroscientific evolution that redefines the relationship between mind, synapses, and recovery.

26.2 Ketamine, the Switch of Hopelessness

Ketamine, an NMDA glutamate receptor antagonist, works in minutes where other antidepressants take weeks. Its mechanism is not "sedative", but synaptic: it stimulates the release of BDNF (brain-derived neurotrophic factor), which promotes the regeneration of neuronal connections.

Indications in bipolarity:

- Resistant depression and mixed phases with severe inhibition.
- Imminent suicidal risk.

Therapeutic effects:

- Mood improvement in 1–2 hours.
- Rapid reduction in suicidal ideation.
- Increased motivation and energy.

Risks:

- Transient dissociation, increased blood pressure, and potential for abuse.

DNP-21-B correlation:

- Normalizes glutamate.
- It increases dopamine and BDNF in a controlled way.

Ketamine doesn't erase sadness —it reminds the brain how to feel hope again.

26.3 Esketamine, the Controlled Evolution of Ketamine

Esketamine (S isomer of ketamine) is administered intranasally under medical supervision. It offers the same antidepressant benefits, but with less dissociation and a better safety profile.

Advantages:

- Quick start (30-60 minutes).
- Suicide risk reduction.
- Controlled application in an outpatient clinic.

Protocol:

- 2 weekly sessions for 4 weeks, then maintenance every 1-2 weeks.
- Always combined with a mood stabilizer.

DNP-21-B:

- Regulates glutamate and dopamine.
- Stimulates frontal neuroplasticity.

Esketamine is the bridge between molecular neuroscience and deep psychotherapy.

26.4 Psilocybin, the Science-Based inner Journey

Psilocybin, derived from psychedelic mushrooms, acts on serotonergic 5-HT2A receptors, resulting in a state of expanded consciousness and high connectivity between neural networks.

Unlike manic euphoria, this state allows for deep emotional reorganization when administered in a guided therapeutic context.

Effects observed:

- Decreased rumination and guilt.
- Increased empathy and self-acceptance.
- Reactivation of vital motivation.

Precautions:

- Risk of triggering hypomania if used without a stabilizer.
- Only under approved clinical protocols and psychotherapeutic accompaniment.

DNP-21-B:

- Increases serotonin and neuroplasticity.
- Default Mode Network.

Psilocybin does not create hallucinations: it reveals neural metaphors for healing.

26.5 ECT, the Electrical Therapy that Saved Thousands of Minds

Electroconvulsive therapy (ECT) has been unfairly stigmatized, but it remains one of the most effective interventions for severe bipolar depression or depression with psychotic symptoms.

It does not destroy neurons: it restores connectivity between hemispheres and normalizes dopaminergic and serotonergic flow.

Indications:

- Resistant depression, catatonia, high suicide risk.

Benefits:

- Clinical response in 80%–90% of severe cases.
- Improved sleep, appetite and motivation.

Side effects:

- Transient confusion, mild loss of recent memory.

ECT is a reset of the brain, not a punishment from the past.

26.6 TMS, Transcranial Magnetic Stimulation

TMS applies magnetic fields to the prefrontal cortex, modulating neuronal excitability without the need for anesthesia or seizures.

Advantages:

- Non-invasive, outpatient and well tolerated.
- Restores synchrony between hemispheres.
- Promotes neuroplasticity and dopaminergic regulation.

Common protocols:

- 20 to 30 sessions, 5 times a week.
- Indicated in bipolar depression and mild mixed phases.

DNP-21-B:

- Balances dopamine and GABA.
- Increases frontal flow and reduces limbic hyperactivity.

TMS doesn't turn off the brain: it reminds you how to think calmly.

26.7 Neuroplasticity and Integrative Psychotherapy

All of these therapies share a common goal: to reopen the neurobiological window of emotional learning. Neuroplasticity, once stimulated, allows psychotherapy, meditation, or art to have a more profound effect. When synapses are regenerated, the soul also finds new paths to heal.

26.8 Science, Mysticism and Hope

The future of bipolar treatment combines biological precision with human depth. It is not just a matter of "activating" the brain, but of integrating mind, emotion and neurochemistry in the same therapeutic symphony. These biological therapies do not replace the doctor or the human bond: they enhance it. The psychiatry of the future will not be based on extinguishing symptoms, but on igniting consciousness (Figure 25).

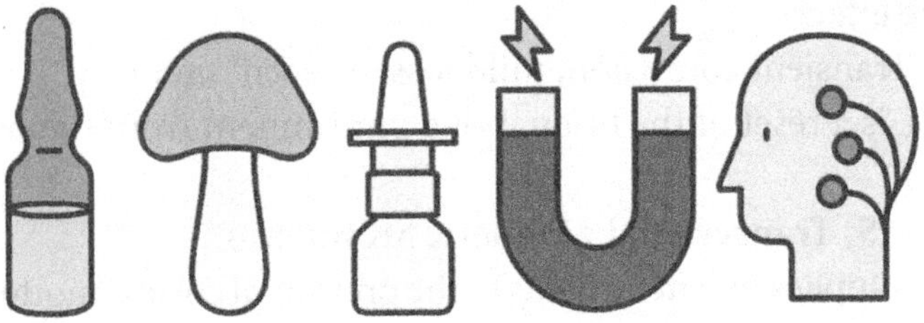

Figure 25. Conceptual illustration of the new biological therapies for bipolar disorder: ketamine, esketamine, psilocybin, transcranial magnetic stimulation and electroconvulsive therapy. It represents the convergence of science, neuroplasticity and hope.

CHAPTER 27
EKG Monitoring, Plasma Levels and Long-Term Security

The science of vigilance: protecting balance while healing.

27.1 To Treat is also to Care

Treatment of bipolar disorder does not end with the prescription. It starts with systematic monitoring, evaluation of side effects, and prevention of metabolic or cardiac complications.

Modern psychiatry understands that emotional stability also depends on physical health, and that proper monitoring turns an effective treatment into a truly safe one. Healing is not only relieving symptoms, but monitoring the systems that sustain life.

27.2 The Heart as a Mirror of Neurochemical Balance

Psychotropic drugs —especially lithium, antipsychotics, and mood stabilizers— can change your heart rate. For this reason, the electrocardiogram (EKG) has become an essential part of modern psychiatric practice.

Most common alterations:

- QT prolongation: associated with quetiapine, ziprasidone or haloperidol.
- Bradycardia or sinus block: possible with lithium.
- Sinus tachycardia: induced by anxiolytics or hypomania.

Clinical recommendations:

- Baseline EKG before starting treatment.
- Repeat when adjusting doses or combining drugs.
- In people over 50 years of age or with comorbidities, perform every 6 months.

Practical interpretation:

- Corrected QT (QTc) > 470 ms in women or > 450 ms in men = high risk.
- In case of prolonged QTc, reduce dose or switch to another drug with less electrical effect.

The EKG doesn't just measure impulses from the heart: it measures the harmony between mind, medicine, and metabolism.

27.3 Monitoring of Plasma Levels

Lithium, valproate, and carbamazepine are narrow-window drugs: too little is ineffective, too much can be toxic.

Table 18 presents the therapeutic ranges, the recommended frequency of plasma control and the main signs of toxicity of the most commonly used mood stabilizers. This provides a practical guide for the safe follow-up and prevention of complications associated with pharmacological treatment.

Table 18. Therapeutic ranges, monitoring, and signs of mood stabilizer toxicity

Medication	Therapeutic range (mEq/L or µg/mL)	Control frequency	Signs of toxicity
Lithium	0.6–1.2 mEq/L	Every 3 months	Gross tremor, diarrhea, confusion, ataxia
Valproate	50–125 µg/mL	Every 6 months	Nausea, weight gain, hepatotoxicity
Carbamazepine	4–12 µg/mL	Every 6 months	Diplopia, ataxia, hyponatremia

Complementary analyses:

- Kidney and thyroid function (lithium).
- Liver enzymes (valproate, carbamazepine).
- Blood count (carbamazepine).

DNP-21-B correlation:

Monitoring allows the identification of subtle neurochemical deviations: altered dopamine or GABA may reflect toxicity or inappropriate dose. The ideal dose is neither the highest nor the lowest: it is the one that respects the patient's physiology.

27.4 Metabolism and Weight Control. The Silent Enemy

Atypical antipsychotics (olanzapine, quetiapine, risperidone) can disrupt appetite and insulin regulation. This leads to metabolic syndrome, characterized by:

- Weight gain.
- Elevated triglycerides.
- Hypertension.
- Insulin resistance.

Recommended monitoring:

- Weight, waist, blood pressure: every 3 months.
- Glucose and lipids: every 6 months.

Protective interventions:

- Regular aerobic exercise.
- Diet rich in fiber, omega-3 and low glycemic index.
- Consider metformin in patients with significant weight gain.

The body also needs mood stabilizers: rest, movement, and nutrition.

27.5 Renal, Hepatic and Thyroid Evaluation

The body's filtering organs reflect the cumulative effect of the treatment.

Kidney (lithium):

- Monitor creatinine and GFR (glomerular filtration rate).
- Avoid dehydration.

Liver (valproate, carbamazepine):

- TGO/TGP control every 6 months.
- Suspend in the event of persistent elevation.

Thyroid (lithium):

- Subclinical hypothyroidism in 10%–15% of patients.
- Requires levothyroxine supplementation.

Biological monitoring protects the patient from the invisible consequences of prolonged treatment.

27.6 Long-Term Security. Beyond Chemistry

Long-term treatment of bipolar disorder is not only measured in plasma levels or EKGs, but also in quality of life.

Your doctor should evaluate:

- Cognitive state and attention.
- Sexual function and motivation.
- Social and labor impact.
- Adherence to treatment.

New biomarkers:

- Salivary cortisol (chronic stress).
- Plasma BDNF (neuronal resilience).
- Heart rate variability (sympathetic-parasympathetic balance).

True safety is not only the absence of toxicity, but the presence of integral well-being.

27.7 Integration of Monitoring into the DNP-21-B Model

DNP-21-B extends classical surveillance by incorporating neurochemical biomarkers along with physiological parameters.

Example of integrated interpretation:

- EKG + dopamine elevated → risk of manic activation.
- High valproate + low GABA → dose adjustment or combined with lamotrigine.
- Low melatonin + high cortisol → circadian stress.

In this way, monitoring becomes a precision medicine tool that personalizes treatment. To watch is to understand the dynamics of the soul through biology (Figure 26).

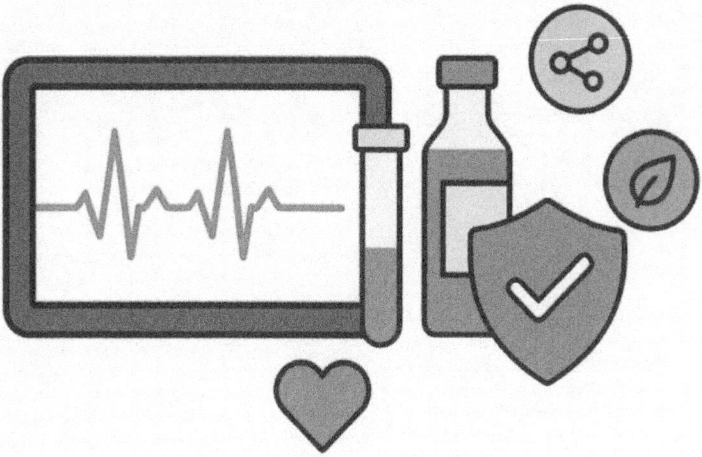

Figure 26. Conceptual representation of medical monitoring in the treatment of bipolar disorder. The illustration reflects the relationship between heart, laboratory and stability. All this symbolizes the balance between mind, medicine and biology.

27.8 The Medicine of Observation

Every EKG, every plasma level, every analysis is a conversation between the body and the psychiatrist. The monitoring doctor listens to the body's whispers before it screams.

Emotional balance is sustained through constant vigilance, clinical empathy, and respect for the patient's physiology. In the art of treating bipolar disorder, follow-up is not bureaucracy: it is compassion in the form of science.

CHAPTER 28
Clinical Algorithms per Phase: Acute Mania, Bipolar Maintenance and Depression

The therapeutic map for navigating the oscillating mind.

28.1 Psychiatry as Dynamic Cartography

Treatment for bipolar disorder cannot be rigid or uniform. Each phase —manic, depressive, mixed, or stability— requires a change in strategy. Clinical algorithms are not automatic prescriptions: they are living maps that guide the doctor from urgency to prevention, adapting to the patient's biochemical and existential rhythm.

Modern psychiatry does not impose stability: it teaches us to find it in the midst of movement. DNP-21-B provides the neurochemical basis for these algorithms, allowing a personalized approach according to the dominant neurotransmitter profile.

28.2 Acute manic phase. Control without shutting down

Therapeutic objectives:

- Reduce dopamine and glutamate.
- Restore sleep and self-control.
- Avoid relapses and hospitalization.

Clinical algorithm:

This algorithm describes a staggered clinical approach for the management of manic or mixed episodes, prioritizing the suspension of destabilizing agents, the establishment of mood stabilizers, the rapid control of acute symptoms, and the consideration of neuromodulatory interventions in refractory cases, with emphasis on safety and clinical monitoring (Table 19).

Table 19. Staggered clinical management of manic or mixed episodes

Step	Intervention	Example or drug	Considerations
1	Discontinue antidepressants	—	Prevents dopaminergic overstimulation
2	Start Mood Stabilizer	Lithium or valproate	Monitor plasma levels
3	Add atypical antipsychotic	Quetiapine, olanzapine or aripiprazole	Rapid control of euphoria and impulsivity
4	Treating insomnia	Lorazepam or melatonin	Do not keep for more than 2–4 weeks
5	Consider TMS or ECT	In refractory cases	Restores cortical connectivity

DNP-21-B correlation:

- Dopamine high → antipsychotic.
- Elevated glutamate → valproate or lamotrigine.
- GABA under → temporary benzodiazepine.

Psychotherapy during mania:

- Brief, focused on limits and containment.
- Avoid deep interpretations during euphoria.

The goal is not to "turn off" the mania, but to give the brain back its ability to brake.

28.3 Bipolar Depressive Phase. Reactivate without Causing a Turn

Therapeutic objectives:

- Raise serotonin and dopamine without overwhelming the system.
- Restore motivation and sleep.
- Avoid antidepressants in monotherapy.

Clinical algorithm:

This algorithm describes the fundamental interventions for the long-term maintenance of bipolar disorder, integrating continuous pharmacological treatment, psychoeducation, circadian rhythm regulation, healthy lifestyle habits and periodic reevaluation of the neurochemical profile using the DNP-21-B model, with the aim of reducing relapses and optimizing functional stability (Table 20).

Table 20. Maintenance Strategy and Relapse Prevention in Bipolar Disorder

Step	Intervention	Example	Considerations
1	Confirm that it is not unipolar depression	DNP-21-B, Medical History	Avoid diagnostic errors
2	Start stabilizer	Lamotrigina or Lithium	Improves affective tone
3	Add antipsychotic with antidepressant effect	Quetiapine or lurasidone	Critical first 2–4 weeks
4	If there is no response, add controlled antidepressant	Bupropion or mirtazapine	Always next to stabilizer
5	Biological alternatives	Ketamine, TMS or ECT	In severe or resistant depression

Psychotherapy during depression:

- Acceptance and commitment therapy (ACT).
- Interventions based on social rhythm.
- Family support and routine reconstruction.

In bipolar depression, lifting your mood without raising dopamine is a clinical art.

28.4 Mixed Phase. When the Soul Accelerates and Shuts Down at the Same Time

The mixed phase is one of the most dangerous: the patient may feel deep sadness and excessive energy, which increases the risk of suicide.

Objectives:

- Balance dopamine and serotonin simultaneously.
- Control impulsivity and emotional dissociation.

Base treatment:

- Valproate or carbamazepine (first options).
- Quetiapine or olanzapine for rapid stabilization.
- Avoid antidepressants; can aggravate agitation.
- Emotional containment psychotherapy.

DNP-21-B correlation:

- High dopamine and glutamate with low GABA → typical mixed pattern.

The mixed mind needs containment more than speed.

28.5 Maintenance Phase. The Real Therapeutic Victory

Objectives

- Prevent manic or depressive relapses.
- Reduce doses without losing stability.
- Rehabilitate cognitive and social functions.

Clinical algorithm:

This algorithm describes the fundamental interventions for the long-term maintenance of bipolar disorder, integrating continuous pharmacological treatment, psychoeducation, circadian rhythm regulation, healthy lifestyle habits, and periodic reevaluation of the neurochemical profile using the DNP-21-B model, with the aim of reducing relapses and optimizing functional stability (Table 21).

Table 21. Maintenance Strategy and Relapse Prevention in Bipolar Disorder

Step	intervention	Treatment	Purpose
1	Maintain mood stabilization	Lithium, lamotrigine or valproate	Therapeutic basis

Step	intervention	Treatment	Purpose
2	Continuing psychoeducation	Individual or familiar	Relapse prevention
3	Sleep control and circadian routine	Melatonin, morning light	Reinforce internal rhythm
4	Physical exercise and a balanced diet	—	Improve metabolism and mood
5	Review DNP-21-B every 6 months	Neurochemical profile	Custom fit

Stability is not a stationary state: it is a regulated dance between neurochemistry, mind and everyday life.

28.6 DNP-21-B Integrative Algorithm

Table 22 presents examples of common neurochemical profiles identified by DNP-21-B, relating them to the most likely clinical phase of bipolar disorder and to suggested therapeutic interventions, which facilitates the translation of mood biology into concrete clinical decisions.

Table 22. Clinical interpretation of DNP-21-B profiles and therapeutic guidance

DNP-21-B Profile	Most likely phase	Suggested Intervention
Dopamine ↑↑ / Glutamate ↑	Mania or mixed	Antipsychotic + valproate
Dopamine ↓ / GABA ↓	Bipolar depression	Lamotrigine + quetiapine
Serotonin ↓ / Cortisol ↑	Anxious depression	Mirtazapine + ACT psychotherapy
GABA ↓ / Melatonin ↓	Bipolar insomnia	Melatonin + sleep hygiene

DNP-21-B translates the biology of mood into concrete clinical decisions.

28.7 Chaos at the Algorithm

The treatment of bipolar disorder is not improvised: it is navigated. Every medical decision, every dose, and every adjustment is part of a dynamic system where science and empathy work together. Algorithms are not a substitute for the doctor; amplify their sensitivity. To treat bipolarity is to teach the brain its own map back home (Figure 27).

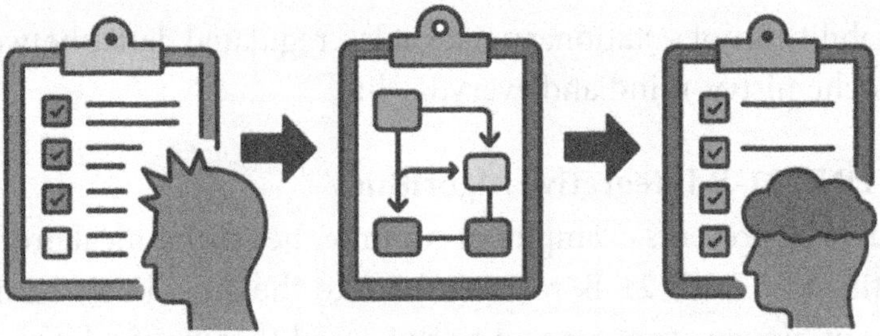

Figure 27. Conceptual representation of clinical algorithms in the treatment of bipolar disorder. Circular trajectories symbolize the transition between mania, depression, and maintenance, reflecting the neurochemical rhythm that guides emotional stability.

PART VI. Non-Pharmacological Interventions

CHAPTER 29
Cognitive-Behavioral Therapy Adapted to Bipolarity

Retrain the mind to re-educate emotion.

29.1 The Mind as a Laboratory of Change

Cognitive behavioral therapy (CBT) has been one of the most effective tools for treating depression and anxiety. However, in bipolar disorder it requires a special adaptation: the bipolar mind not only feels intensely, but also thinks extremely. The challenge is not to eliminate negative or euphoric thoughts, but to recognize their cyclical patterns and learn to respond rather than react.

CBT does not seek to control the emotion, but to teach the patient to converse with it without fear. The goal is to transform the cognitive distortions typical of bipolar disorder into more stable, flexible, and realistic thoughts, strengthening the sense of identity and self-control.

29.2 Neurocognitive Basis of Bipolar Thinking

In bipolarity, the prefrontal circuits responsible for logical reasoning and planning are temporarily dominated by the limbic systems of impulse and emotion.

During mania, thinking accelerates, self-perception is distorted, and a sense of omnipotence appears. In depression, those same circuits are inhibited, giving rise to thoughts of worthlessness, guilt, or hopelessness.

The therapist helps the patient recognize cognitive biases that change with the mood phase:

- Mania: overvaluation of abilities, denial of risk, magical thinking.
- Depression: excessive self-criticism, catastrophic thinking, irrational guilt.
- Mixed phase: alternation between grandiosity and despair.

Understanding bipolar thinking is like observing the emotional climate of the brain: there are storms, but also sunrises.

29.3 Core Tools of Adapted CBT

1. **Automatic Thought Recording:**

The patient learns to write down thoughts that arise at critical moments and analyze them according to evidence and emotion.

2. **Cognitive challenge:**

It is taught to question extreme thoughts through Socratic questions:

- "What evidence do I have that this is completely true?"
- "Could there be another, more balanced explanation?"

3. **Behavioral restructuring:**

Daily micro-actions are established that promote habits of stability (schedules, sleep, exercise, food, social contact).

4. **Relapse prevention:**

The patient identifies early signs of mood changes (decreased sleep, increased energy, ideas of greatness) and develops an action plan to intervene in time.

5. **Use of DNP-21-B in psychotherapy:**

The neurochemical profile helps to personalize cognitive strategies:

- High dopamine → work impulsivity and control immediate pleasure.
- Low serotonin → reinforce gratitude, compassion, and patience.
- Under GABA → teach relaxation and mindful breathing.

The brain learns not only with medicines, but with deliberate thought and re-educated emotion.

29.4 Clinical Example

Patient: 32 years old woman, diagnosed with bipolar II. During hypomanic phases, he starts multiple work projects that he abandons weeks later. In the depressive phase, she feels incapable and self-destructive.

In therapy, you learn to identify your "all or nothing" pattern and create a scale from 1 to 10 to measure the intensity of your ideas before you act.

Results:

- Reduction of impulsive behaviors.
- Greater continuity in projects.
- Recovery of self-esteem based on real actions, not emotional states.

The patient did not lose her creativity: she learned to give it direction (Figure 28).

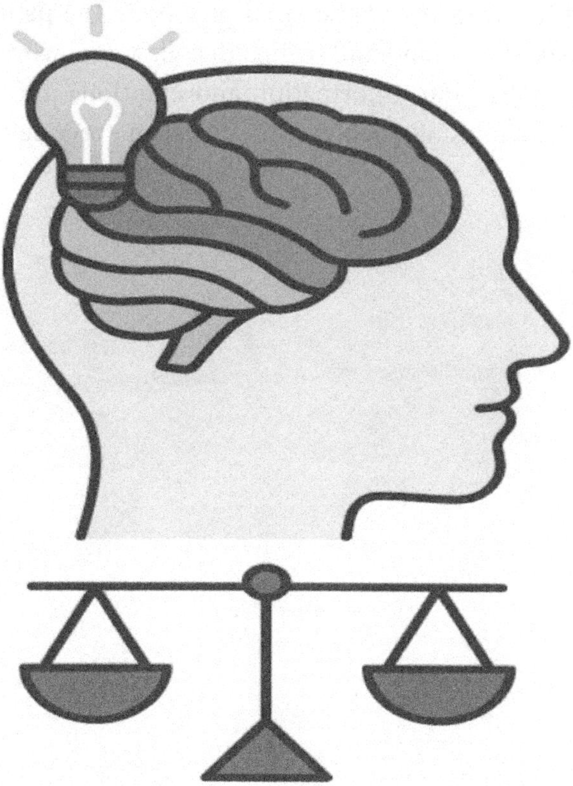

Figure 28. Conceptual representation of cognitive-behavioral therapy in bipolar disorder. The geometric lines reflect the reorganization of thought and the integration between emotion and reason as a path to stability.

29.5 Integration of CBT with Other Therapies

CBT is enhanced when combined with:

- Family psychoeducation: helps detect signs of early change.
- Interpersonal and social rhythm therapy (IPSRT): maintains schedules and routines.
- Mindfulness and acceptance: reduces emotional reactivity.

Each tool reinforces the same principle: awareness and self-control as pillars of bipolar balance.

29.6 Thinking with Tenderness and Discipline

CBT adapted to bipolar disorder teaches that thinking can be an anchor in the midst of the swell of mood. The patient stops fighting against his mind and begins to collaborate with it, transforming impulses into information and emotions into wisdom. Thought is the invisible medicine that is taken every day.

CHAPTER 30
Individual and Family Psychoeducation

Turning knowledge into prevention and understanding.

30.1 Educating to Stabilize

Psychoeducation is much more than explaining a diagnosis: it is teaching how to live with it. In bipolar disorder, knowledge transforms uncertainty into strategy and fear into cooperation.

When the patient and their family understand how the disorder works, relapses decrease, adherence improves, and communication becomes more empathetic. Information does not cure, but it illuminates the path to stability.

Individual and family psychoeducation turns the patient into an active agent of their treatment, and the family environment into a system of therapeutic support, not of surveillance or judgment (Figure 29).

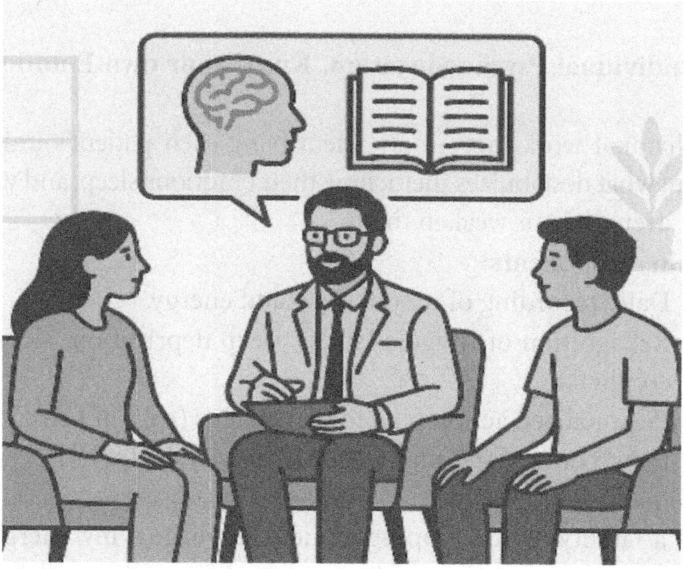

Figure 29. Conceptual representation of individual and family psychoeducation in bipolar disorder. The image symbolizes communication, shared learning, and empathic understanding between patient, therapist, and family.

30.2 Objectives of Bipolar Psychoeducation

1. **Understanding the disorder:**
   Identify symptoms, phases, triggers, and personal patterns of relapse.
2. **Promote therapeutic adherence:**
   Explain how medications work and the consequences of stopping them.
3. **Develop preventive strategies:**
   Establish routines, monitor sleep, and recognize early warning signs.
4. **Strengthen the family network:**
   Teach family members to respond with empathy and without confrontation.
5. **Reduce stigma:**
   Replace guilt with knowledge and shame with scientific understanding.

Understanding bipolar disorder is not labeling the person, but freeing them from the fear of their own mind.

30.3 Individual Psychoeducation. Know your own Emotional Map

Individual work focuses on identifying each patient's unique pattern: what destabilizes them, how their emotions sleep, and what habits strengthen or weaken them.

Main components:

- Daily recording of mood, sleep and energy.
- Recognition of triggers (stress, sleep deprivation, alcohol, conflicts).
- Personalized action plan for early signs (e.g., "if I sleep less than 5 hours for 2 nights, notify the psychiatrist").

The patient learns to see his mood as an observable variable, not as a fatality. By developing clinical language ("my energy is high but my judgment is stable"), you become an active collaborator with your mental health team. When the patient understands his own pattern, he stops fearing the cycle.

30.4 Family Psychoeducation. Allies Instead of Judges

The family environment can be the greatest support or the greatest stressor of the bipolar patient. Therefore, educating the family is part of the treatment.

Objectives:

- Understand that mood swings are not "attitudes", but neurochemical processes.
- Promote nonviolent communication and empathy.
- Teach how to spot signs of relapse:
  - Persistent speech acceleration or irritability.
  - Progressive isolation or excessive fatigue.
  - Impulsive spending, grandiose projects, or ideas of futility.

Strategies:

- Regular therapeutic meetings with the patient and their family.
- Training in active listening and crisis management.
- Clarification of limits: support without invading.

The educated family becomes the best mood stabilizer. The patient learns to view their mood as an observable variable, not as something inevitable. By developing clinical language ("my energy is high but my judgment is stable"), they become an active collaborator with their mental health team. When patients understand their own patterns, they stop fearing the cycle.

30.5 The DNP-21-B Model Applied to Psychoeducation

The DNP-21-B provides a biological dimension that reinforces family understanding::

- It allows you to visualize which neurotransmitters predominate in each phase.
- It explains why certain behaviors (hyperactivity, insomnia, sadness) are not voluntary, but chemical expressions.
- It facilitates empathy based on science: the patient does not "choose" their oscillation, but they can learn to manage it.

Example of use:

A mother observes that her son has a phase of intense irritability. By reviewing your DNP-21-B profile, you understand that your dopamine and glutamate are elevated. Instead of arguing, he decides to promote rest, avoid excessive stimuli and accompany with serenity. Understanding the neurochemistry of the loved one turns love into a clinical tool.

30.6 Group Dynamics and Educational Resources

In many mental health centers, psychoeducational workshops are organized where patients and families learn together.

Frequently Asked Topics:

- What to do in the event of a relapse?
- How to talk to the doctor?
- Sleep and self-care strategies.
- Myths about medication.

These dynamics foster community and reduce social isolation, one of the greatest enemies of stability.

30.7 Knowing is Caring

Psychoeducation teaches that the bipolar mind is not an enemy, but a sensitive system that needs constant understanding. Knowledge transforms family coexistence into an act of therapeutic collaboration.

The educated patient is empowered; the informed family protects without judging; and the doctor accompanies more effectively. Educating is not only explaining: it is offering a compass to those who cross the sea of the soul.

CHAPTER 31
Interpersonal and Social Rhythm Therapy

Retrain the brain's emotional clock.

31.1 Time as Medicine

Interpersonal and social rhythm therapy (IPSRT) was developed by Ellen Frank and her team at the University of Pittsburgh to treat bipolar disorder. Its objective is not only to improve human relationships, but also to synchronize emotional life with the biological clock.

In bipolar disorder, cycles of sleep, eating, work, and relationships directly influence mood. IPSRT teaches the patient to regulate these rhythms and maintain a constant balance, which reduces relapses and improves functional stability. Mood depends not only on what we feel, but also on when and how we live.

31.2 Biological and Emotional Foundations of Social Rhythm

The bipolar brain has a circadian vulnerability: its internal clocks —regulated by melatonin, cortisol and dopamine— can be easily desynchronized by external factors (travel, stress, time changes, conflicts).

When this happens, the limbic system becomes uncoordinated with the prefrontal, which generates alterations in energy, sleep and emotions. The IPSRT proposes to align the internal clock with everyday life, adjusting the social rhythm (schedules, interactions, activities) to individual biology.

Example:

A patient who works at night and sleeps irregularly may present with mixed or recurrent depressive symptoms. Treatment would include reorganizing their daily routine, regulating meals, and re-educating the sleep-wake cycle. Reordering time is a silent way of reordering the mind.

31.3 Structure of the IPSRT

The therapy is divided into four complementary phases:

a) Evaluation phase

The therapist identifies the patient's life rhythms, key relationships, and life events that disrupt their emotional stability.

Instruments:

- Daily sleep, activity, and mood log.
- Interpersonal pattern analysis.
- Social Rhythm Metric questionnaires.

b) Intervention phase

The therapist and the patient establish concrete objectives to stabilize routines:

- Maintain fixed schedules for sleeping, eating and working.
- Reduce stimuli before sleeping.
- Balance social life without excesses.

c) Interpersonal phase

We work on relational conflicts, unresolved grief or role changes (marriage, maternity, retirement). The patient learns communication and problem-solving strategies.

d) Maintenance phase

Over time, the patient develops natural self-regulation. Learn to identify their early warning rhythms and restructure them before they cause a relapse. The IPSRT does not only teach how to sleep well: it teaches how to live in tune with one's own biological clock.

31.4 Neurochemical Intervention: the Link between Rhythm and Neurotransmission

Table 23 describes the relationship between the different phases of the circadian rhythm, the predominant neurotransmitters at each moment of the day and their associated neuroemotional functions. The importance of biological synchronization in mood stability and affective regulation is highlighted. Each biological rhythm modulates the release of neurotransmitters.

Table 23. Circadian rhythm, dominant neurotransmitters, and neuroemotional functions

Rhythm	Dominant neurotransmitter	Function
Deep sleep	GABA, melatonine	Recovery, emotional consolidation
Morning	Dopamine, cortisol	Energy, concentration
Afternoon	Serotonin	Well-being, stability
Night	GABA, Melatonine	Deactivation of the limbic system

DNP-21-B complements IPSRT by identifying which neurotransmitters are out of phase and which habits stabilize them.

For example:

- Patients with nocturnal high dopamine → avoid screens and caffeine.
- Low evening serotonin → light physical activity in the evening.

Each neurotransmitter follows its own rhythm. The therapist teaches you to listen to it.

31.5 Clinical Example

Pacient: 40 years old man, diagnosed with bipolar I, with relapses after work shift changes.

Problem: sleep disturbances, morning irritability, social isolation.

Treatment:

- Circadian routine adjustment.
- Weekly IPSRT sessions focused on family conflicts.
- Complementary use of melatonin and morning light therapy.

Result:

- Improved sleep and energy.
- Reduction of mixed episodes.
- Greater interpersonal stability.

When the body and emotions beat at the same rate, the mind rests.

31.6 IPSRT as a Bridge between Science and Everyday Life

The IPSRT unites biology and humanity. It treats the patient not as a set of symptoms, but as a rhythmic organism, in constant interaction with its environment. It promotes discipline without rigidity, structure without repression and freedom with responsibility. Balance is not imposed: it is synchronised.

31.7 The Melody of Inner Time

Interpersonal and social rhythm therapy teaches that each person has a unique "emotional tempo". Respecting it is a form of preventive medicine. The therapist acts as an orchestra conductor who helps the patient to rediscover his harmony between the rhythms of the body, mind and human relationships. To heal is to learn to play the music of one's own clock (Figure 30).

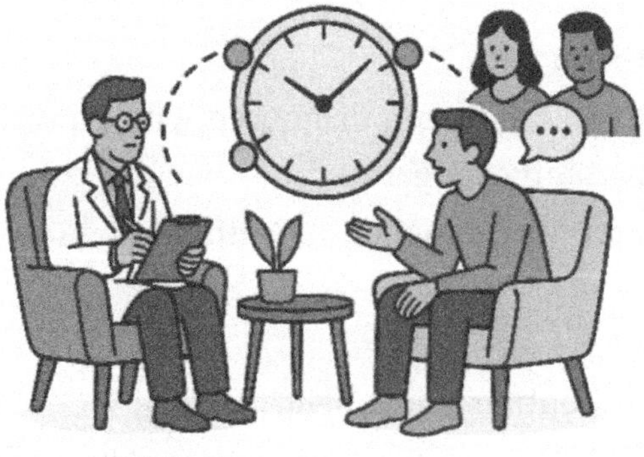

Figure 30. Conceptual representation of interpersonal therapy and social rhythm (IPSRT). The image symbolizes the synchronization between time, emotions and human relationships as an axis of stability in bipolar disorder.

CHAPTER 32
Acceptance and Commitment Therapy (ACT) and DBT

Accept to transform: the mind as an ally, not as an enemy.

32.1 From Control to Conscious Acceptance

Bipolar disorder puts human beings in front of a paradox: the more they try to control their emotions, the more they overflow. Acceptance and commitment therapy (ACT) and dialectical-behavioral therapy (DBT) offer a different approach: it is not about eliminating suffering, but about learning to relate to it differently. Overcontrol makes you sick; Intelligent acceptance liberates.

ACT and DBT teach the bipolar patient to accept their inner experience, develop conscious presence, and act on their values, even when mood fluctuates. They do not seek to "cure" bipolarity, but to broaden consciousness and strengthen psychological flexibility.

32.2 Acceptance and Commitment Therapy (ACT): Living in Coherence

The ACT is based on a central principle: human suffering does not come from having negative thoughts, but from fighting against them. In bipolarity, this struggle manifests itself in the fear of relapse, guilt for past episodes or denial of the disease.

Main objectives:

1. Acceptance: stop fighting with emotions.
2. Cognitive defusion: observing thoughts without identifying with them.
3. Contact with the present: reduce rumination and fear of the future.
4. Personal values: identifying what gives meaning to life beyond mood.

5. Committed action: acting consistently with those values, even in difficult times.

Clinical example:

A patient with bipolar II disorder is afraid to start a new relationship for fear of losing control. In therapy, she learns to recognize that thought ("I might become unstable") as a phrase, not a prophecy. He decides to act on his value of emotional connection, not on fear. Accepting is not giving up, it is stopping running away from oneself.

32.3 Dialectical Behavioural Therapy (DBT): Balance between Reason and Emotion

DBT, developed by Marsha Linehan, was originally created for borderline disorder, but its dialectical approach is extremely useful in managing impulsivity, emotional reactivity, and suicidal behavior in bipolar.

Its central philosophy is the dialectic between acceptance and change: the therapist teaches the patient that he or she can accept his or her suffering and, at the same time, work to modify it.

Main components:

1. Mindfulness: observe without judging.
2. Emotional regulation: identifying and modulating intense emotions.
3. Tolerance to discomfort: learning to resist the impulse without acting destructively.
4. Interpersonal effectiveness: communicating needs without aggression or submission.

Clinical example:

A patient in the mixed phase feels like self-harm. Using DBT techniques, you learn how to apply the "stop and breathe" exercise before acting, and how to call your therapist or use a crisis plan. Over time, their tolerance for discomfort increases, and the attacks decrease in frequency. DBT does not suppress emotions, it teaches you to navigate between them without sinking.

32.4 Neurobiology of Emotional Acceptance and Regulation

The continuous practice of mindfulness and acceptance activates the medial prefrontal cortex and the anterior cingulate, regions related to emotional regulation and empathy.

Simultaneously, it decreases the hyperactivity of the amygdala, reducing the intensity of manic or depressive reactions.

DNP-21-B correlation:

- Acceptance reduces cortisol and norepinephrine.
- Mindfulness increases serotonin and GABA.
- Committed action stimulates balanced dopamine and sustained motivation.

Emotional neuroplasticity is strengthened when we stop resisting and start observing.

32.5 ACT + DBT Integration in Bipolar Treatment

Combined, ACT and DBT form a powerful therapeutic framework:

- ACT teaches you to live with emotional oscillation without running away.
- DBT teaches how to regulate that oscillation with compassion and structure.

Example of integration:

During a phase of irritability, the patient practices mindfulness (DBT) to reduce emotional intensity, and then applies cognitive defusion (ACT) to avoid identifying with thoughts of guilt or frustration.

This approach unites Eastern wisdom of mindfulness with Western scientific precision. Serenity does not come when emotions disappear, but when we learn to breathe them.

32.6 Acceptance as an Inner Revolution

ACT and DBT invite the patient to stop living at war with their own mind. Instead of forcing stability, they cultivate an attitude of gentle observation and emotional discipline.

The result is not perfection, but functional peace: the ability to feel without overflowing, to act without losing direction, and to heal without denying the complexity of life. Acceptance does not cure bipolarity, but it teaches the soul to coexist with it in peace (Figure 31).

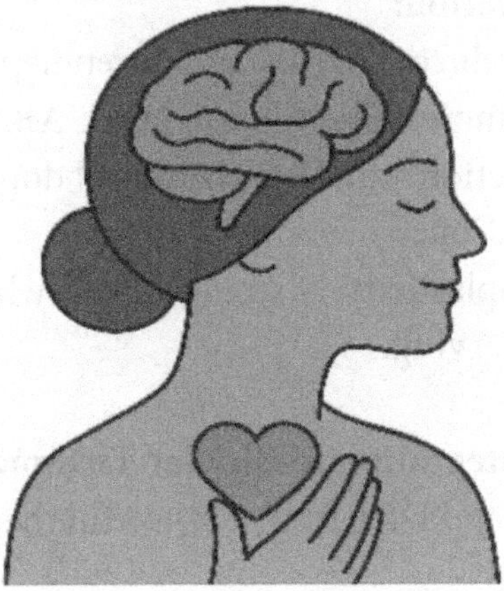

Figure 31. Conceptual representation of acceptance and commitment therapy (ACT) and DBT. The image symbolizes the conscious mind, self-compassion, and committed action as guides to emotional healing.

CHAPTER 33
Mindfulness, Meditation and Mind-Body Techniques

Re-educate the nervous system from calm.

33.1 The Body as an Entrance to the Mind

In the treatment of bipolar disorder, drugs stabilize the chemistry, psychotherapy organizes the thoughts, but the body is the door that connects both dimensions.

Mindfulness practices, meditation, and mind-body techniques (such as mindful breathing, yoga, tai chi, or progressive muscle relaxation) act directly on the brain-body axis, balancing the systems that regulate emotion, sleep, and attention.

Calm is not imposed by reason: it is trained from the body. These techniques help the bipolar patient to recognize the present moment, to decrease the physiological reactivity of the amygdala and to reconnect with the feeling of internal stability, even when the environment or mood is altered.

33.2 Mindfulness: Full Attention without Judgment

Mindfulness is not an exotic Eastern technique, but a trained form of awareness. It consists of observing thoughts, sensations and emotions without reacting immediately to them. Its objective is not to empty the mind, but to inhabit it with serenity.

In bipolarity, where thoughts can be fast, intrusive, or painful, mindfulness allows the patient to create space between emotion and action.

Basic exercise:

- Sit with your eyes closed.
- Observe the breath for one minute.
- Mentally name thoughts ("worry", "memory", "plan") without trying to eliminate them.

Mindfulness does not stop the storm, but it teaches us to observe it without being shipwrecked.

Studies show that regular mindfulness practice lowers cortisol levels, improves sleep, and strengthens the prefrontal cortex, helping to prevent relapses.

33.3 Meditation: The Neuroscience of Silence

Meditation, in any of its variants (guided, transcendental, compassionate or concentrative), modulates the circuits of attention, empathy and emotional regulation.

During practice, the flow of thoughts slows down, the heart rate stabilizes, and the mind enters a state of neurophysiological coherence.

Proven neurobiological changes:

- Decreased activity of the amygdala.
- Increased cortical thickness in anterior cingulate regions.
- Greater connectivity between the insula and the orbitofrontal cortex (centers of body awareness and emotional regulation).

Clinical example:

A patient with episodes of hypomania practices 10 minutes of compassionate meditation each morning. After three months, he reports less irritability and better control of impulsivity. Inner silence is not empty, it is a laboratory of self-regulation.

33.4 Body-Mind Techniques: Physiology of Stability

a) Diaphragmatic breathing

It decreases the activation of the sympathetic system and activates the vagus nerve, inducing relaxation. Exercise: inhale 4 seconds, hold 4, exhale 6, hold 2.

b) Progressive muscle relaxation

Tense and release each muscle group. It improves body perception and reduces tension accumulated in phases of anxiety or agitation.

c) Therapeutic yoga and tai chi

It combines conscious movement and rhythmic breathing. It increases the production of GABA and serotonin, which promotes a natural neurochemical balance.

d) Biofeedback and neurofeedback

They train the patient to self-regulate their brain waves or heart rate through visual feedback, which strengthens body self-awareness. The educated body becomes the best mood stabilizer (Figure 32).

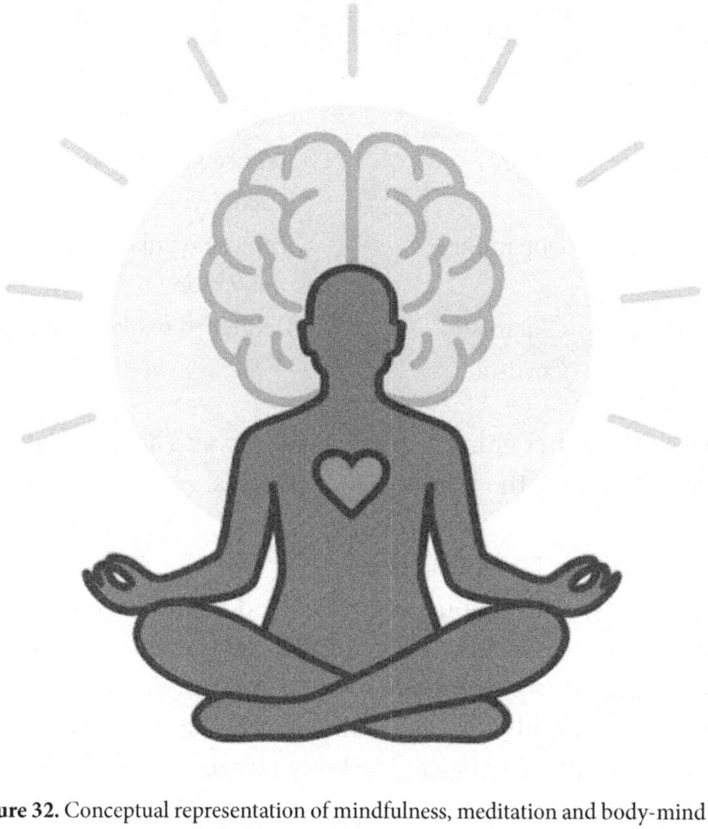

Figure 32. Conceptual representation of mindfulness, meditation and body-mind techniques. The calm figure symbolizes conscious breathing, the connection between body and mind, and the inner balance achieved through daily practice.

33.5 Integration with the DNP-21-B Model

The DNP-21-B allows us to observe how mind-body practices modulate specific neurotransmitters.

Table 24 relates different mind-body practices with the main neurotransmitters involved and their therapeutic effects on emotional regulation, stress control and mood stability, highlighting their value as complementary interventions within a comprehensive approach to bipolar disorder.

Table 24. Mind-Body Practices and Their Therapeutic Neurochemical Impact

Practice	Key Neurotransmitter	Therapeutic effect
Meditation	Serotonin	Improved well-being and emotional stability
Mindful breathing	GABA	Reduced anxiety and reactivity
Yoga / tai chi	Dopamine	Impulse regulation and motivation
Mindfulness	Glutamate / Cortisol	Decreased oxidative stress

These techniques enhance brain plasticity and act as a natural adjuvant therapy in the prevention of relapses.

33.6 Serenity as a Daily Practice

Mindfulness meditation and body-mind techniques teach the bipolar patient that emotional stability is not a destination, but a daily training. Every conscious breath, every moment of mindfulness, or every body stretch is a therapeutic act that reorganizes the brain's circuits of balance. The body remembers the calm that the mind forgets.

CHAPTER 34
Social Support, Psychoeducational Groups and Rehabilitation Programs

Healing in company: the therapeutic force of the community.

34.1 Stability as a Collective Construction

Bipolar disorder is a condition that is often experienced in solitude. However, studies and clinical experience show that human connection is one of the most potent mood stabilizers.

Social support, psychoeducational groups, and psychosocial rehabilitation programs not only improve adherence to treatment, but also provide meaning, belonging, and hope. Loneliness aggravates symptoms; The conscious company softens them.

The goal of this part of treatment is not only to keep the patient functional, but to reintegrate them into life with healthy bonds, meaningful activities, and a network of emotional and professional support.

34.2 The Clinical Value of Social Support

Social support works as a buffer against stress. Interaction with family, friends, therapists or peers reduces emotional overload and improves self-regulation. Scientific evidence shows that patients with strong social networks have:

- Fewer hospitalizations.
- Shorter and less severe episodes.
- Better adherence to pharmacological treatment.
- Greater sense of vital purpose.

Clinical example:

A patient who lives alone and rarely socializes shows frequent relapses. By joining a weekly psychoeducational group, he begins to improve his communication, organizes his routine and regains the motivation to work. No medication can replace the feeling of being heard and understood.

34.3 Psychoeducational Groups. Learning in Community

Psychoeducational groups combine the teaching of clinical knowledge with the construction of social and emotional skills. They are led by a professional (psychiatrist, psychologist or occupational therapist) and are organised into thematic modules (Table 25).

Table 25. Fundamental components of a psychoeducation program in bipolar disorder

Module	Contents	Objective
Education about the disorder	What is bipolar? Symptoms, phases, prevention	Understanding and acceptance
Adherence and medication	Types of drugs, effects, myths	Responsible use
Early Signs and Relapses	Pattern Identification	Early intervention
Stress and self-care	Mind-body strategies, sleep, eating	Functional stability
Family communication	Assertiveness and limits	Healthy relationships

The group dynamic allows each participant to learn from the experience of the other. Listening to similar stories decreases guilt and normalizes the emotional experience. Psychoeducational groups are laboratories of empathy and emotional learning.

34.4 Psychosocial Rehabilitation Programmes

Rehabilitation programs have a more comprehensive approach. They seek to restore the patient's functionality in all areas: work, cognitive, interpersonal and spiritual.

Typical Components:

- Social skills training.
- Memory, attention and organization workshops.
- Employment guidance and support for economic reintegration.
- Recreational activities and artistic expression.

Many centers also include mindfulness, music therapy or art therapy workshops, in which creativity is encouraged as a therapeutic tool.

Example:

A community rehabilitation program in Spain incorporated gardening and therapeutic cooking activities. Patients reported increased self-esteem, improved concentration, and reduced depressive symptoms. To recover is to participate in life again, not just to avoid relapse.

34.5 Integration with the DNP-21-B

DNP-21-B provides a neurochemical framework for personalizing social support and rehabilitation. Table 26 relates different neurochemical profiles with recommended psychosocial approaches, guiding daily and therapeutic interventions that complement pharmacological treatment and favor the patient's emotional and functional self-regulation according to the DNP-21-B model.

Table 26. Psychosocial interventions according to neurochemical profile (DNP-21-B model)

Neurochemical profile	Recommended approach
High dopamine	Structured activities that channel energy (sports, art projects)
Low serotonin	Emotional support groups, compassion therapy, and volunteering
GABA deficiency	Training in relaxation, yoga, mindfulness

Neurochemical profile	Recommended approach
Glutamatergic alteration	Cognitive programs and sensorineural stimulation

In this way, rehabilitation becomes a practical extension of neurochemical balance.

34.6 The Role of the Family and Community Environment

Families and communities can become true therapeutic networks if they receive adequate education and support. In Mexico, Spain and the United States there are associations and NGOs that accompany patients in processes of labor integration, legal advice and psychological guidance. Recovery does not happen in isolation, but in dialogue with the world.

34.7 Healing in the Plural

Treatment for bipolar disorder does not end at the doctor's office. It requires community, purpose, and meaningful bonding. Every conversation, every gesture of support, every group that shares experiences is part of an invisible medicine: human connection.

The stable bipolar is not the one who lives without crisis, but the one who has learned to ask for help before falling (Figure 33).

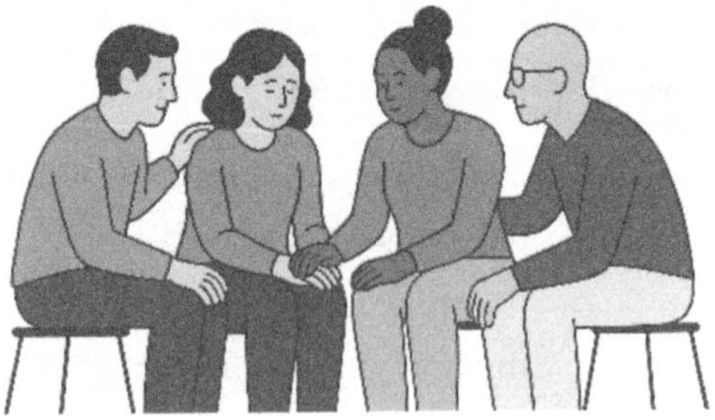

Figure 33. Conceptual representation of social support and psychoeducational groups. The image reflects empathy, listening and accompaniment as essential elements.

PART VII.
The Impact on Life

CHAPTER 35
Bipolar Disorder at Work, Studies and Professional Life

Balance productivity, purpose, and mental health.

35.1 The Challenge of Functioning in a World that does not Stop

Work and studies are an essential part of human identity. They give us purpose, structure, and belonging. However, for people with bipolar disorder, these settings can become sources of both fulfillment and risk.

Mood swings can interfere with focus, productivity, or work relationships; but with the right strategies, it's possible to maintain a stable and meaningful career without sacrificing mental health. Job stability is not measured by the absence of crises, but by the ability to prevent them and face them with awareness.

35.2 Challenges of the Work and Academic Environment

Bipolar disorder affects three critical dimensions of performance:

1. Cognitive: difficulty concentrating, remembering information, or making decisions under pressure.
2. Emotional: sudden changes in mood, irritability or social withdrawal.
3. Physical: sleep disturbances, irregular energy, fatigue or hyperactivity.

In highly competitive work or study environments, these symptoms can lead to guilt, perfectionism, or fear of stigma, increasing the risk of relapse.

Clinical example:

An engineer with bipolar I disorder has a hypomanic phase during a major project. He works 16 hours a day, sleeps little and ends up with a severe depressive episode. In therapy, learn to set boundaries and schedule strategic breaks. The prevention of burnout (burnout syndrome) is also relapse prevention.

35.3 Strategies for Job and Academic Stability

1. Structured routine: maintain consistent sleep, meal, and work schedules.
2. Dosed tasks: divide projects into small and realistic stages.
3. Transparent communication: inform a trusted supervisor or advisor about the condition if necessary.
4. Pause: use brief breathing or mindfulness techniques during the day.
5. Symptom monitoring: record changes in energy, irritability or concentration.

Emotional self-discipline is a form of professional intelligence.

35.4 Reasonable Accommodations in the Work or Study Environment

Legislation in many countries, such as the Americans with Disabilities Act (ADA) or the General Law for the Inclusion of Persons with Disabilities in Mexico, protects the right to request reasonable accommodations. These do not imply privileges, but conditions that favor healthy performance.

Examples of useful accommodations:

- Flexible schedules in phases of therapeutic adjustment.
- Quiet spaces or partial remote work.
- Clear feedback and support in task organization.
- Avoid night shifts or excessive working hours.

Adapting the environment is not a weakness: it is clinical intelligence applied to real life.

35.5 Emotional Education in the Professional Field

The professional success of the bipolar patient does not depend only on medical treatment, but also on emotional education and self-awareness. Learning to recognize early signs (such as increased energy or decreased sleep) can prevent crises without interrupting productivity.

Therapeutic exercise:

Create a "job stability map", identifying:

- Activities that generate well-being.
- Destabilizing factors (stress, conflicts, excess stimuli).
- Regulation strategies (active rest, breathing, social support).

Work ceases to be a threat when it becomes a space of conscious balance.

35.6 The DNP-21-B Model Applied to Professional Performance

DNP-21-B can be used to identify the predominant neurochemical profile and design appropriate work strategies. Table 27 offers practical guidelines for the professional environment based on the DNP-21-B neurochemical profile with the aim of optimizing performance, preventing emotional overload and promoting sustainable work functioning aligned with the individual's neurobiological needs.

Table 27. Professional recommendations according to DNP-21-B neurochemical profile

DNP-21-B Profile	Professional recommendation
High dopamine	Avoid task overload; Prioritizing focus and rest
Low serotonin	Promote recognition, collaborative work and spaces of gratitude
GABA deficiency	Include short breaks and relaxation techniques
Glutamatergic alteration	Reduce multitasking, prioritize simple projects

Understanding the neurochemistry of one's work allows you to maintain productivity without losing stability.

35.7 Redefining Success

Success in bipolar disorder is not measured by accumulating achievements, but by maintaining coherence between well-being and purpose. With treatment, support and self-knowledge, the patient can develop a fulfilling career, without sacrificing their authenticity or their health. It is not a question of being perfect, but of being sustainable (Figure 34).

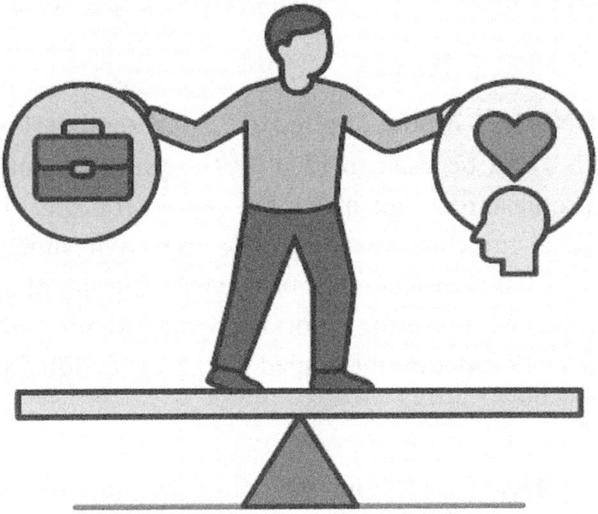

Figure 34. Conceptual representation of the balance between professional life and mental health in bipolar disorder. The figure symbolizes the search for harmony between productivity, purpose, and emotional well-being.

CHAPTER 36
Affective Relationships, Family and Emotional Conflict Management

Loving without losing balance: conscious bonds in bipolarity.

36.1 Love as a Mirror of the Mind

Affective relationships are one of the most challenging and beautiful dimensions of life. In bipolar disorder, these relationships become especially complex because mood can change the way you love, communicate, and perceive the other.

During mania, love can feel like limitless expansion; during depression, like an unfillable void. But between the two extremes there is a real space where it is possible to build stable, authentic and deeply human bonds. Loving with bipolarity is not impossible; it is to love with awareness, self-care and healthy limits.

36.2 How do Bipolar Phases Affect Relationships?

Emotional oscillations impact couple, family, and social dynamics in different ways:

- **Manic or hypomanic phase:**
  Excessive energy, impulsivity, hypersexuality, excessive expenses or need for attention. The couple may feel displaced or confused.
- **Depressive phase:**
  Withdrawal, loss of interest, low self-esteem, hopelessness. The other may interpret these symptoms as heartbreak or rejection.
- **Mixed phase:**
  Irritability, emotional contradiction and chaotic communication. Avoidable conflicts and ruptures are generated if there is no understanding of the cycle.

Clinical example:

A woman in the hypomanic phase starts multiple projects and becomes extremely sociable, which generates insecurity in her partner. In therapy, both learn to recognize early signs and establish preventive agreements. Prevention as a couple is just as important as individual medical treatment.

36.3 Conscious and Emotionally Safe Communication

The bipolar heart needs clear, paused, and empathetic language. Intense arguments or prolonged misunderstandings can amplify emotional swings.

Keys to healthy communication:

1. Speak in moments of calm, never during a crisis.
2. Describe feelings, not accuse ("I feel confused" instead of "you never understand me").
3. Avoid generalizations ("always", "never", "everything").
4. Recognize one's own emotions before responding.
5. Agree on a "time-out" when someone feels they are going to lose control.

Therapeutic exercise:

Each partner writes how they perceive the other's mood swings and how they can offer support without losing their own well-being. Communication is the most powerful emotional stabilizer within a relationship.

36.4 Family: Allies, Not Judges

The family environment often witnesses emotional ups and downs. Education and understanding of the disorder are essential to avoid dynamics of guilt, overprotection or excessive criticism.

Recommendations for families:

1. Learn to differentiate voluntary behavior from symptom.
2. Do not respond with anger or sarcasm during unstable phases.
3. Participate in family therapy or support groups.
4. Also take care of the caregiver's mental health.

An informed family can be as therapeutic as the best drug (Figure 35).

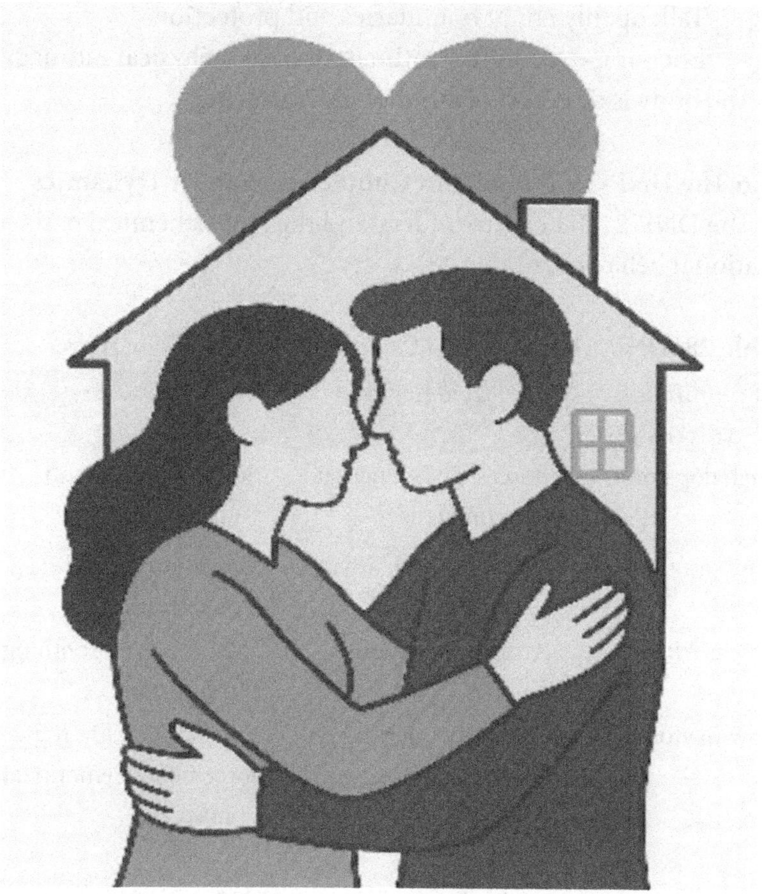

Figure 35. Conceptual representation of affective relationships and emotional connection in bipolar disorder. The figures symbolize empathy, communication, and shared healing among those who learn to love with awareness.

36.5 Sexuality and Intimate Ties

During the manic or hypomanic phases, there may be an increase in sexual desire, search for new experiences or risky behaviors. In depression, the opposite: loss of interest and disconnection. It is vital to approach sexuality without guilt or taboos, integrating it into the therapeutic plan.

Keys:

- Recognize hypersexuality as a symptom, not as a moral trait.

- Talk openly about boundaries and protection.
- Encourage emotional intimacy, not just physical intimacy.

The body is also part of emotional treatment..

36.6 The DNP-21-B Model in Couple and Family Dynamics

The DNP-21-B helps to understand the neurochemical basis of relational behaviors (Table 28).

Table 28. DNP-21-B Model in Couple and Family Dynamics

Predominant neurotransmitter	Typical behavior	Therapeutic strategy
High dopamine	Impulsivity, seduction, overconfidence	Set boundaries and routines
Low serotonin	Irritability, sensitivity to rejection	Gratitude and validation exercises
Low GABA	Anxiety, constant tension	Breathing and soothing physical contact
Low oxytocin	Difficulty bonding or trusting	Couples therapy, reinforcement of emotional contact

Understanding the biology of the bond helps to forgive what chemistry alters.

36.7 Loving from Inner Stability

Relationships in the context of bipolar disorder require emotional maturity, constant communication, and deep self-knowledge. When both parties understand that the disorder does not define the person, but is part of their emotional landscape, love ceases to be a battlefield and becomes a territory of shared growth. The most stable love is not the one that avoids storms, but the one that learns to navigate with awareness and tenderness.

CHAPTER 37
Sexuality, Impulsivity and Self-Esteem

The body as a mirror of the spirit and the inner bond.

37.1 Desire in an Oscillating Brain

Sexuality in bipolar disorder is a direct expression of the neurochemical state. During manic or hypomanic phases, craving may intensify to become impulsive; in depressive phases, it may disappear completely. This seesaw generates confusion, guilt and relational difficulties, both in life as a couple and in the perception of one's own body.

Desire is not an enemy of balance; it needs to be understood, not repressed. Talking about sexuality in psychiatry does not mean talking only about pleasure or behavior, but about identity, bonding and self-esteem. Integrating this topic into clinical evaluation allows us to prevent risky behaviors, promote conscious intimacy and restore a healthy relationship with one's own body.

37.2 The Neurochemistry of Desire

Table 29 summarizes the main neurotransmitters involved in mood regulation, describing their central neuropsychological function and the clinical manifestations associated with their excess or deficit in bipolar disorder, which facilitates an integrated understanding between neurobiology and symptomatology. Sexual desire depends on a delicate balance between neurotransmitters and hormones.

Table 29. Main neurotransmitters involved in bipolarity and its clinical manifestations

Neurochemical	Main function	Excess or deficit in bipolarity
Dopamine	Initiative, pleasure, motivation	Excess → hypersexuality; Deficit → anhedonia

Neurochemical	Main function	Excess or deficit in bipolarity
Serotonin	Impulse regulation, emotional connection	Deficit → impulsivity and risk-seeking
GABA	Inhibitory control and inner soothing	Deficit → disinhibition and anxiety
Oxytocin	Attachment and trust	Deficit → difficulty in establishing stable bonds

During mania, the brain enters a state of dopaminergic overstimulation. Sensations are amplified, judgment is weakened, and desire can become risky behavior. In depression, the opposite happens: libido decreases and the body is perceived as alien. Sexual balance is not achieved by controlling the body, but by understanding the mind that inhabits it.

37.3 Hypersexuality and Behavioral Risk

Hypersexuality is one of the most common symptoms of the manic or mixed phase. It manifests as increased sex drive, multi-partner searching, compulsive pornography, or excessive spending on erotic experiences. It is not a sign of immorality, but a clinical expression of neurochemical lack of control.

Clinical example:

A 42 years old man with bipolar I disorder reports that, during his manic phases, he feels an "unstoppable sexual energy" and acts impulsively, which damaged his marriage. After starting treatment with lithium and psychoeducation, he learns to recognize the early signs and stop climbing.

Therapeutic recommendations:

- Include hypersexuality in the management plan.
- Set behavioral and financial boundaries.

- Promote body awareness exercises and self-control techniques.
- Involve the partner or sex therapist in the process.

The control of impulse is not born of repression, but of self-knowledge.

37.4 Depression, Body and Self-Esteem

During bipolar depression, the body may feel heavy, dull, or "lifeless". The loss of sexual desire is mixed with guilt, shame and a sense of worthlessness, which affects self-esteem. The patient may emotionally distance themselves from their partner or even avoid physical contact for fear of rejection.

Recovery techniques:

- Somatic re-education (yoga, breathing, conscious touch).
- Body acceptance therapy.
- Gradual resumption of affective and sexual contact.
- Avoid judging desire as an indicator of personal worth.

Reconnecting with the body is reconnecting with life (Figure 36).

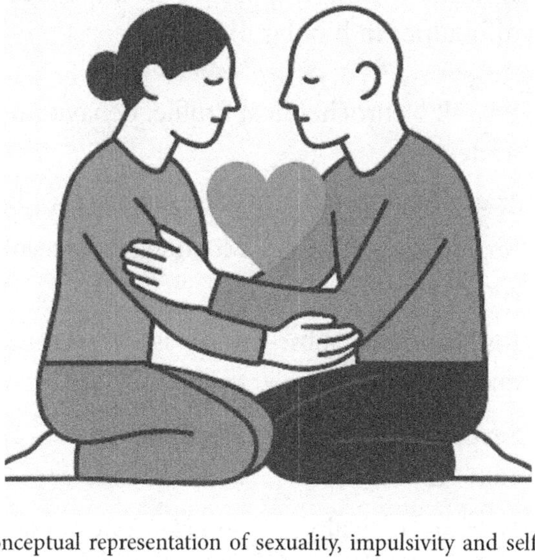

Figure 36. Conceptual representation of sexuality, impulsivity and self-esteem in bipolar disorder. The shapes and colors symbolize the emotional energy that oscillates between desire, control, and self-connection.

37.5 Self-Esteem and Conscious Sexuality

The bipolar cycle can erode self-esteem due to impulsive behaviors or subsequent self-criticism. However, it can also become an opportunity to reconstruct sexual and emotional identity from compassion.

Helpful Practices:

- Body gratitude journal (recognizing pleasurable sensations without judgment).
- Guided visualization of the body as a safe space.
- Relearning pleasure from calm, not from euphoria.

Healthy sexuality is born when desire ceases to be an escape and becomes presence.

37.6 Integration with the DNP-21-B Model

The DNP-21-B allows the identification of the predominant neurochemical profile that influences sexual and emotional behavior. Table 30 relates different neurochemical profiles identified by the DNP-21-B model with specific behavioral risks and suggested therapeutic intervention strategies, which facilitates a preventive and clinically sensitive approach to impulsive behaviors and bonding difficulties in bipolar disorder.

Table 30. DNP-21-B Neurochemical Profile, Behavioral Risks, and Intervention Strategies

DNP-21-B	Main risk	Suggested Intervention
High dopamine	Impulsivity and sexual addiction	Mood stabilizer regulation
Low serotonin	Risk behaviors, subsequent guilt	Compassion and mindfulness therapy
GABA deficiency	Sexual anxiety, difficulty relaxing	Breathing exercises and mind-body techniques
Low oxytocin	Isolation, difficulty with attachment	Stimulate safe physical contact and emotional connection

Understanding the biochemistry of desire frees you from guilt and guides you toward a more conscious sexuality.

37.7 The Reconciled Body

Sexuality in bipolar disorder should not be feared, but rather integrated as an essential part of the balancing process. The therapeutic goal is not to extinguish desire, but totransform it into a force for connection, creativity, and self-acceptance. The body is not the enemy of the bipolar mind; it is its wisest ally when it is listened to with respect.

CHAPTER 38
Bipolar Disorder and Addictions: Common Comorbidities

When the brain seeks balance in the external.

38.1 Two Disorders That Are Enhanced

The relationship between bipolar disorder and addictions is deep and bidirectional. Between 40 and 60% of patients with bipolar disorder develop, at some point in their lives, an addiction to substances such as alcohol, cannabis, cocaine, stimulants or anxiolytic drugs.

Both conditions share common neurobiological mechanisms, such as dopaminergic dysfunction, impulsivity, and the need to regulate extreme emotions. Addictions are not born of pleasure, but of the desperate attempt to anesthetize pain or prolong euphoria.

Substance use may seem like temporary relief at first, but it ends up exacerbating bipolar symptoms, interfering with treatments, and increasing the risk of hospitalization or suicide.

38.2 Why is the Bipolar Brain more Vulnerable to Addictions?

The brain's reward system, regulated by dopamine, GABA, and glutamate, is hypersensitive in bipolarity. During mania, the search for pleasure intensifies; During depression, the mind seeks to escape the void. Both directions lead to the same point: loss of impulse control.

Vulnerability factors:

- Shared genetic inheritance.
- Need to self-regulate intense emotions.
- Low tolerance for frustration.
- Easy access to substances during expansive episodes.
- Stigmatization or lack of adequate treatment.

The bipolar patient does not seek the drug: he seeks rest from the internal chemical imbalance.

38.3 Substances most Associated with Bipolar Disorder

Table 31 summarizes the perceived initial effects of different psychoactive substances and the main risks associated with their use in people with bipolar disorder, highlighting their potential to destabilize mood, induce relapse, and complicate the clinical and therapeutic course.

Table 31. Psychoactive substances and clinical risks in bipolar disorder

Substance	Initial effect	Main risk
Alcohol	Sedation, anxiety relief	Nervous system depressant; aggravates depressive phases
Cannabis	Relaxation, mild euphoria	Psychosis, disorganization, hypomania
Cocaine/ stimulants	Energy, self-confidence	Triggers mania and paranoia
Benzodiazepines	Reduced anxiety and insomnia	Dependence, severe withdrawal
Opioids	Analgesia, emotional calm	High addiction, respiratory depression

The pattern is clear: immediate relief is paid for with a greater imbalance of mood and neurochemistry.

Clinical example:

A patient with bipolar II disorder resorts to alcohol to "lower his mind" during hypomanic episodes. Over time, you develop dependency and increase your risk of severe depression. By starting dual therapy (addiction + bipolar), she manages to sustain her abstinence for more than a year.

38.4 Dual Diagnosis and Integrated Treatment

The concept of dual disorder recognizes the coexistence of mental illness and addiction. The approach must be integrated, simultaneous and multidisciplinary in order to avoid treating only one of the problems.

Elements of dual treatment:

1. Complete psychiatric evaluation with history of use.
2. Pharmacological intervention adjusted to both conditions.
3. Individual and group psychotherapy.
4. Psychoeducation and relapse prevention.
5. Family and community support network.

There is no emotional sobriety without neurochemical sobriety.

38.5 Recommended Therapeutic Strategies

- Lithium or valproate: stabilize mood and reduce impulsivity associated with craving.
- Atypical antipsychotics: control psychotic or mixed symptoms.
- Naltrexone or acamprosate: help reduce alcohol consumption.
- Cognitive-behavioral and motivational therapies: strengthen awareness of illness.
- Mindfulness and body-mind techniques: reduce stress and increase self-regulation.

Therapeutic exercise:

Ask the patient to draw their "emotional timeline", marking when the consumption began and what they were trying to relieve. This exercise usually reveals the emotional root of the habit.

38.6 Integration with the DNP-21-B Model

Table 32 relates different neurochemical profiles identified by the DNP-21-B model with frequently associated addiction patterns and the main therapeutic intervention strategies, offering a clinical framework for the integrated approach to bipolar and substance use disorders.

DNP-21-B allows correlating each type of addiction with a specific neurochemical imbalance:

Table 32. Psychoactive substances and clinical risks in bipolar disorder

DNP-21-B	Associated addiction	Main intervention
High dopamine	Cocaine, stimulants	Regulation with lithium, mindfulness
Low serotonin	Alcohol, compulsive behaviors	Compassion and structure psychotherapy
GABA deficiency	Benzodiazepines	Gradual substitution and relaxation training
Glutamatergic dysfunction	Cannabis, hallucinogens	Cognitive rehabilitation and pharmacological stabilization

All addiction is a form of imperfect self-medication; treatment seeks to replace it with conscious regulation (Figure 37).

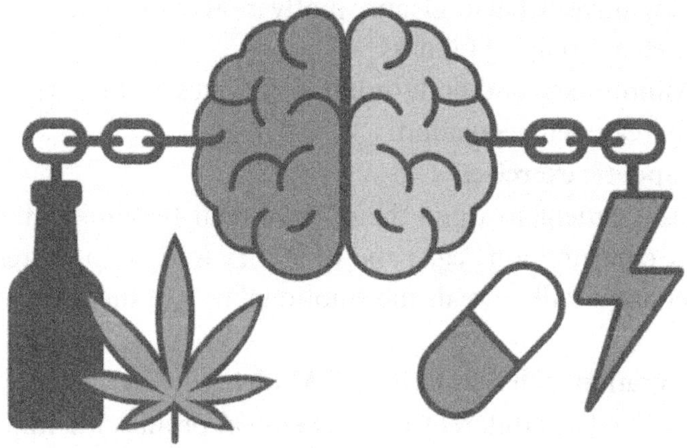

Figure 37. Conceptual representation of the comorbidities between bipolar disorder and addictions. The image symbolizes the neurochemical connection between both disorders and the release process towards recovery.

38.7 Regaining Control Without Losing Hope

Bipolarity and addiction are two languages of the same brain trying to heal. The path to recovery is not about repressing desire, but about transforming the search for pleasure into the search for balance. With comprehensive treatment, support, and self-compassion, it's possible to live without relying on substances or inner chaos. True sobriety is not abstaining, but reconnecting with life.

CHAPTER 39
Suicide Risk: Assessment, Prevention and Accompaniment

To listen to the silence before the abyss.

39.1 Suicide as an Expression of Invisible Suffering

Suicidal risk in bipolar disorder represents one of the greatest clinical and human challenges of modern psychiatry. It is estimated that up to 20% of patients with bipolar disorder die by suicide, and about 50% have attempted suicide at least once. This risk is not a sign of weakness or unwillingness, but the consequence of extreme neurochemical dysregulation combined with hopelessness, guilt, and emotional exhaustion.

Suicide is not a desire to die, but a desperate desire to stop suffering. Talking about suicide with the patient does not increase the risk; on the contrary, it opens a space of containment, empathy and therapeutic possibility.

39.2 Neurobiology of Suicidal Drive

The suicidal act arises from a complex interaction between neurotransmitters, brain networks and psychological factors.

In bipolar disorder, three central mechanisms stand out:

- Serotonin deficiency: decreases impulse control and resilience.
- Dopaminergic dysfunction: causes anhedonia and loss of vital motivation.
- HPA axis hyperactivity (stress): raises cortisol, which causes agitation and insomnia.

Added to this are alterations in the prefrontal cortex (judgment and decision-making) and the amygdala (processing of fear and guilt). The person does not rationally "choose" to die; His brain, saturated by pain, loses the ability to visualize alternatives. Hopelessness is both a neurochemical and an emotional disturbance.

39.3 Risk Factors and Warning Signs

Biographical factors:

- Previous history of suicide attempts.
- Family history of suicide.
- Diagnosis of bipolar I with mixed or severe depressive episodes.
- Alcohol or drug use.
- Chronic medical illnesses or persistent pain.

Behavioral signs:

- Isolation or sudden dismissals.
- Give away meaningful personal items.
- Phrases of despair ("I can't stand it anymore", "it would be better to disappear").
- Sudden mood swings, especially sudden improvement after deep depression.
- Abandonment of treatment.

The highest risk does not always occur in sadness, but at the moment when the patient recovers enough energy to act.

39.4 Clinical Assessment of Suicide Risk

All psychiatric consultations should include a structured assessment of suicide risk, especially in depressive or mixed phases.

Useful tools:

- Columbia-Suicide Severity Rating Scale (C-SSRS).
- Beck Scale for Suicide Ideation (BSSI).
- Patient Health Questionnaire (PHQ-9)–ítem 9.
- DNP-21-B: allows correlating neurochemical imbalances with suicidal vulnerability.

Key Clinical Interview:

- Explore ideas of death or hopelessness.
- Evaluate the presence of plan, method, and access.
- Inquire about protective factors (family, faith, purpose, treatment).
- Classify the risk as mild, moderate, or severe.
- Develop a personalized security plan.

Assessing risk is not guessing the future: it is building a bridge between crisis and hope.

39.5 Prevention and Management Strategies

- Hospitalization when there is an imminent risk or loss of judgment.
- Continuous monitoring during the first weeks after discharge.
- Pharmacological adjustment: lithium, quetiapine and lurasidone have been shown to reduce suicidal ideation.
- Psychotherapy focused on crisis and emotional regulation.
- Family intervention and training in early detection.
- Restriction of lethal force in the home.

Clinical example:

A 28 years old woman with bipolar II disorder presents with recurrent suicidal ideation. A "life plan" is worked out together with your therapist: emergency numbers, contact persons, meaningful activities, and daily reminders of purpose. Preventing suicide is accompanying the mind while it finds reasons to stay.

39.6 The Role of Lithium and Neuroprotection

Among all mood stabilizers, lithium is the only one with solid evidence in suicide prevention. It works by modulating serotonin, decreasing impulsivity, and restoring neuronal connectivity. Its sustained use reduces suicide risk by up to 60%, even in patients with previous attempts. Lithium doesn't just stabilize the mood, it protects life.

39.7 Integration with the DNP-21-B Model

Table 33 relates different neurochemical profiles of the DNP-21-B model with predominant emotional vulnerabilities and suggested therapeutic approaches, integrating pharmacological, psychotherapeutic and somatic interventions for a sensitive and personalized clinical approach to bipolar disorder. The DNP-21-B allows the identification of the neurochemical profile of greater suicidal vulnerability and the guidance of personalized interventions.

Table 33. DNP-21-B Profiles, Emotional Vulnerabilities, and Therapeutic Approaches

DNP-21-B	Main vulnerability	Therapeutic approach
Low serotonin	Impulsivity, hopelessness	Lithium, psychotherapy, mindfulness
Baja dopamina	Anhedonia, lack of purpose	Behavioral Activation and gratitude
Glutamate excess	Anxiety, insomnia, agitation	Stabilizers and body-mind techniques
GABA deficiency	Fear, chronic tension	Somatic intervention, breathing, family support

Each neurotransmitter can be a point of fragility or a gateway to recovery.

39.8 Hope as a Treatment

Suicide is not fought only with medication, but with presence, listening and meaning. The empathetic accompaniment of the therapist, the family and the community transforms despair into possibility. Talking about pain with respect and without judgment not only saves lives: it restores human dignity. Suicide prevention begins when someone dares to listen without fear (Figure 38).

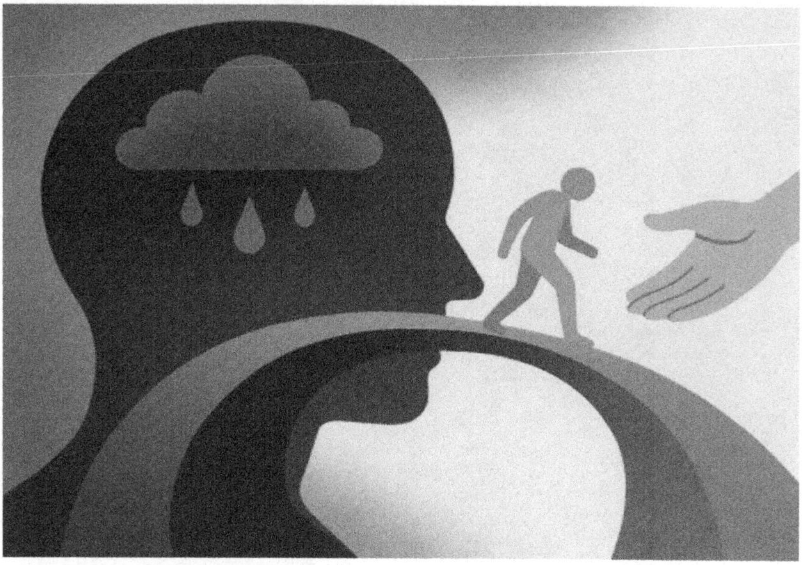

Figure 38. Conceptual representation of suicide risk and prevention in bipolar disorder. The light that emerges from above symbolizes empathy, hope, and the therapeutic power of human connection in the face of pain.

CHAPTER 40
Crisis, Hospitalizations and Emergency Management

When the mind overflows: act calmly in the face of chaos.

40.1 The Crisis as a Turning Point

In the course of bipolar disorder, acute crises —whether manic, depressive, or mixed—represent moments of profound disorganization, both for the patient and for his or her environment.

During these episodes, the person may lose the ability to self-care, judgement or connect with reality, sometimes requiring hospitalisation or immediate intervention.

The crisis is not the end of the therapeutic path, but an opportunity for restart and learning. Proper crisis management is one of the most important clinical competencies to ensure safety, stability, and long-term recovery.

40.2 Early Identification of a Crisis

Seizures rarely come on suddenly. They are usually announced by prodromal symptoms that can be recognized with training and attention.

Warning signs:

- Decreased sleep without tiredness.
- Increased energy or irritability.
- Accelerated speech or flight of ideas.
- Impulsive behaviors or excessive spending.
- Disinterest, withdrawal, or thoughts of death.
- Distrust, agitation or delusional ideation.

Early recognition of these signs by the patient, family, or clinical team dramatically reduces the need for hospitalization. Crisis prevention begins with awareness of one's own body and mind (Figure 39).

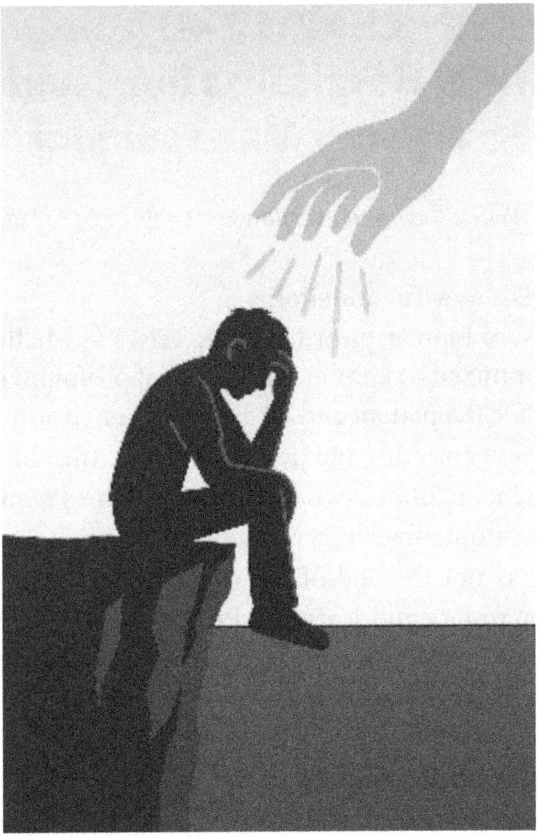

Figure 39. Conceptual representation of the crisis and therapeutic accompaniment in bipolar disorder. The hand that descends symbolizes the professional and human help that guides the patient from the abyss of imbalance to emotional stability.

40.3 Clinical Evaluation During Emergency

In a crisis situation, the first step is to ensure the safety of the patient and the environment. The psychiatrist or emergency team should conduct a structured evaluation that includes:

1. Level of awareness and orientation.
2. Presence of suicidal, homicidal, or psychotic ideation.
3. Adherence to treatment and recent substance use.
4. Recent stressors (grief, breakups, conflicts).
5. Medical conditions that may aggravate symptoms.

In psychiatric emergencies, acting calmly and empathetically is just as important as medication.

40.4 Hospitalization: when and why?

Hospitalization should not be understood as a punishment, but as a temporary therapeutic resource to restore neurochemical and emotional stability.

Main indications:

- Suicidal risk or aggressiveness.
- Severe psychotic episodes.
- Dangerous or impulsive behaviors.
- Lack of family or social support.
- Failure of outpatient treatment.

During hospitalization, the goal is to protect, stabilize, and reintegrate. Treatment includes intensive pharmacotherapy, psychoeducation and discharge planning. Entering does not mean going backwards, but stopping to regain one's balance.

40.5 Emergency Management at Home or Consultation

Many mild or moderate seizures can be managed outside the hospital if you have a structured action plan.

Key elements of the crisis plan:

- Identify early signs of relapse.
- Contact the psychiatrist or therapist before the crisis escalates.
- Avoid important decisions (moving, breakups, large purchases).
- Reduce stimuli (noise, light, arguments).
- Initiate breathing or mindfulness techniques.
- Maintain a safe and supervised environment.

Clinical example:

A patient with a history of mixed episodes notices increasing irritability and difficulty sleeping. Together with his family, he activates his "personal protocol": rest, caffeine suspension and immediate contact with his doctor. This prevents a complete relapse. Having a crisis plan is like having a map before the storm hits.

40.6 Emergency and Containment Drugs

During an acute crisis, medications may be needed to stabilize the patient quickly.

Common Options:

- Benzodiazepines (lorazepam, clonazepam): reduce agitation and make it easier to sleep.
- Atypical antipsychotics (olanzapine, haloperidol, ziprasidone): control mania or psychosis.
- Intravenous/oral lithium or valproate: stabilize mood progressively.

Use should always be temporary and supervised by a professional, prioritizing safety and clinical monitoring. Emergency medication is not a substitute for treatment, it only protects you while balance is restored.

40.7 Integration with the DNP-21-B Model

DNP-21-B allows seizures to be anticipated by identifying individual neurochemical patterns.

Table 34 relates the different neurochemical profiles of the DNP-21-B model with the most likely types of seizures in bipolar disorder and the recommended preventive strategies, which allows anticipating decompensations and strengthening clinical stability through timely and personalized interventions.

Table 34. DNP-21-B Profiles, Likely Crisis Types, and Preventive Strategies

DNP-21-B Profile	Most likely type of crisis	Preventive strategy
High dopamine	Mania or impulsivity	Structured routine, sleep, stabilizers
Low serotonin	Depression and hopelessness	Psychotherapy, mindfulness, social support
Glutamate Excess	Mixed states or severe anxiety	Breathing techniques, GABAergics
GABA Deficiency	Agitation, insomnia	Exercise, relaxation, biofeedback

Each neurochemical profile has its Achilles' heel, but also its door to prevention.

40.8 From Crisis to Growth

Every crisis can be transformed into a lesson in self-knowledge. With adequate treatment, family accompaniment and preventive tools, the patient learns to recognize imbalance patterns and act before collapse. A mind that learns from its crises becomes its own refuge.

PART VIII. Integrative and Holistic Approaches

CHAPTER 41
Physical Exercise and Mental Health in Bipolar Disorder

Moving the body to stabilize the mind.

41.1 The Body as a Natural Stabilizer of Mood

For a long time, physical exercise was considered only a lifestyle recommendation; today we know that it is a therapeutic intervention with a neurobiological basis.

In bipolar disorder, movement doesn't just strengthen the body: it regulates neurotransmitters, improves sleep, reduces anxiety, and acts as a natural modulator of the dopaminergic and serotonergic axis.

Moving is not running away from pain, but transforming it into useful energy for healing. Exercise can be as effective as a drug in preventing relapse, as long as it is practiced with consistency, awareness and clinical accompaniment.

41.2 Neurochemical Effects of Exercise

Each session of physical activity stimulates the release of dopamine, serotonin, endorphins and BDNF (brain-derived neurotrophic factor), substances that promote neuroplasticity and neuronal repair.

Specific Benefits:

- Dopamine: improves motivation and mental clarity.
- Serotonin: stabilizes mood and decreases irritability.
- GABA: reduces physiological anxiety.
- Endorphins: generate a feeling of well-being.
- BDNF: stimulates synaptic regeneration and protects against relapses.

Every movement is a synapse that awakens.

41.3 Recommended Types of Exercise for Bipolar Patients

Table 35 summarizes the main types of physical exercise recommended in bipolar disorder, their orientation frequency and the associated therapeutic benefits, highlighting the role of body movement as a modulator of mood, sleep and emotional regulation within a comprehensive approach.

Table 35. Physical Exercise, Recommended Frequency, and Therapeutic Benefits in Bipolar Disorder

Type of exercise	Frequency	Main benefit
Aerobic (walking, swimming, biking)	4-5 times/week	Regulates mood and improves sleep
Strength Training	2-3 times/week	Increases dopamine and self-confidence
Yoga o taichí	2-4 times/week	Increases GABA and reduces cortisol
Mindful running or mindful walking	Daily	Promotes emotional regulation

Clinical example:

A 45 years old patient with bipolar II initiates a 30-minute morning walking program. After 6 weeks he improves his energy, his sleep and manages to reduce the need for benzodiazepines.

41.4 The Risk of Excess: Exercise and Mania

In some patients, excessive practice can become a trigger for hypomanic or manic episodes. Too much exercise stimulates dopamine and adrenaline at levels similar to those of an expansive state.

Risk indicators:

- Compulsive or prolonged training (>2 hours a day).
- Denial of tiredness or injuries.
- Decreased sleep without fatigue.
- Euphoria or irritability after exercise.

Discipline heals; the compulsion sickens. Balance is about keeping exercise as a medicine, not a leak.

41.5 Integration of Exercise into the Therapeutic Plan

Exercise should be integrated as part of the multidimensional treatment of bipolar disorder, along with pharmacotherapy, psychotherapy, and psychoeducation.

Practical strategy:

1. Assess clinical status: avoid intense exercise during acute episodes.
2. Set realistic goals: gradual frequency and medical supervision.
3. Record progress: Use of journals or apps.
4. Include social accompaniment: walking with family members or groups.
5. Integrate the DNP-21-B: use the neurochemical profile to choose the most beneficial type of exercise.

Table 36 links the different neurochemical profiles of the DNP-21-B model with recommended types of physical exercise and their expected effects, which facilitates a personalized physical activity prescription aimed at mood regulation, stress reduction and emotional stability.

Table 36. Physical exercise recommendations according to DNP-21-B neurochemical profile

DNP-21-B Profile	Recommended Exercise	Expected Effect
High dopamine	Yoga, breathing	Mental calm
Low serotonin	Outdoor hike	Emotional well-being
GABA Deficiency	Swimming, tai chi	Deep relaxation
Glutamate excess	Gentle stretches	Decreased stress

The body becomes a laboratory of chemical balance when it moves with purpose.

41.6 Movement as Medicine of the Soul

Physical exercise is one of the most accessible and profound forms of emotional regulation. Each step, breath, or stretch helps synchronize the mind with the body, transforming chaotic energy into inner harmony. The bipolar mind finds its rhythm when the body moves again with awareness (Figure 40).

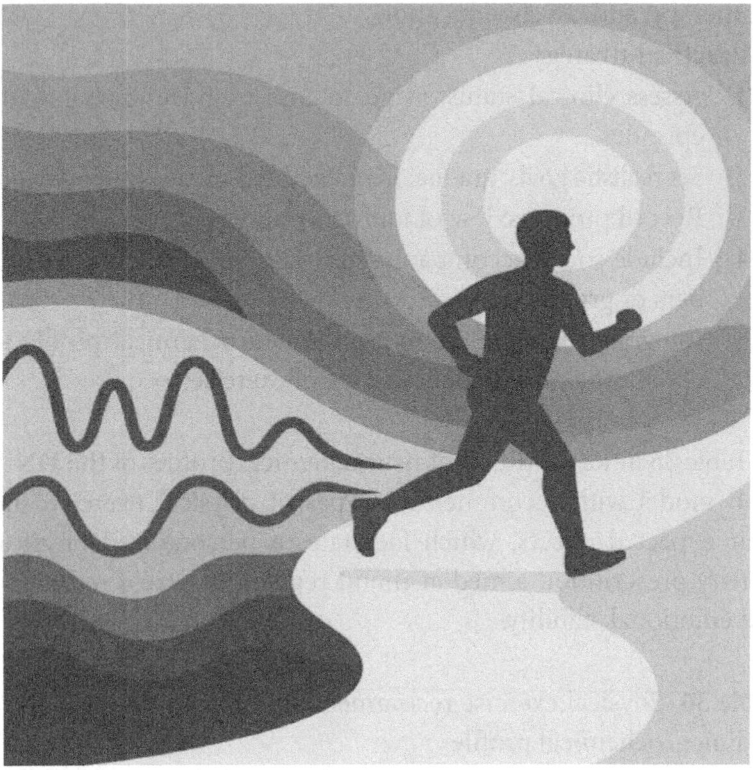

Figure 40. Conceptual representation of physical exercise as a therapeutic tool in bipolar disorder. The light waves surrounding the body symbolize neurochemical regulation, energy balance, and the mind-body connection achieved through conscious movement.

CHAPTER 42
Nutrition, Inflammation and Brain Microbiota

Mental health is also cooked in the gut.

42.1 The New Frontier of Nutritional Psychiatry

Over the past two decades, science has confirmed a profound relationship between diet, inflammation, and mental health. The gut, far from being an isolated organ, functions like a second brain: it contains millions of neurons, produces neurotransmitters such as serotonin, and constantly communicates with the central nervous system through the gut-brain axis.

Eating well not only fuels the body, but also emotional stability. In bipolar disorder, a pro-inflammatory diet can aggravate mood episodes, while a balanced diet helps reduce relapses, improve energy, and optimize response to medications.

42.2 Brain Inflammation and Dysfunction

Modern research shows that bipolar disorder is associated with a chronic low-grade inflammatory state, characterized by elevated levels of cytokines such as IL-6, TNF-α, and ultrasensitive CRP.

These substances alter mitochondrial function and synaptic plasticity, interfering with neurotransmitters such as dopamine and serotonin.

Clinical consequences:

- Higher frequency of mixed episodes.
- Persistent fatigue and mental fog.
- Decreased neuroplasticity.
- Worse response to pharmacological treatment.

The swollen brain does not think clearly or feel steadily.

42.3 The Gut Microbiota: an Ecosystem that Influences Mood

More than 100 trillion bacteria live in the human instinct, which make up the intestinal microbiota. This ecosystem regulates the production of serotonin, dopamine, GABA, and short-chain fatty acids, which directly impact brain function (Figure 41).

Factors that damage the microbiota:

- Antibiotics and ultra-processed diets.
- Refined sugar and trans fats.
- Chronic stress and sleep deprivation.

Factors that strengthen it:

- Diet rich in fiber, fruits and vegetables.
- Natural fermented products (kefir, yogurt, kimchi).
- Omega-3, prebiotics and probiotics.

Taking care of the intestinal flora is taking care of the neurochemistry of the soul.

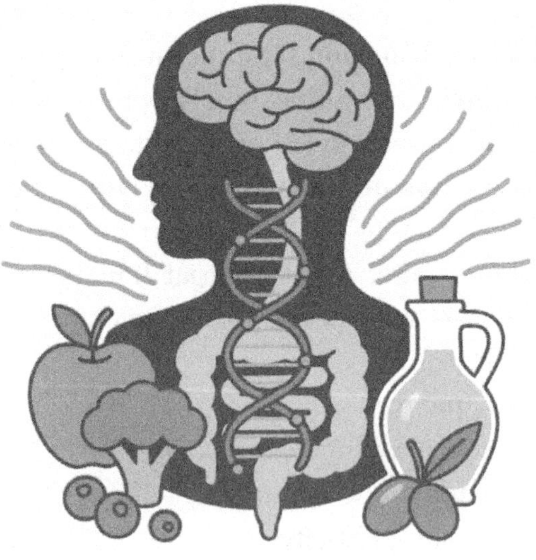

Figure 41. Conceptual representation of nutrition, inflammation, and the gut-brain connection in bipolar disorder. The figure illustrates how healthy foods and a balanced microbiota influence brain function and emotional stability.

42.4 Nutrients that Protect the Bipolar Brain

Table 37 summarizes the main nutrients with evidence of benefit in brain health and mood regulation in bipolar disorder. Its food sources and therapeutic effects are indicated, emphasizing the role of nutrition as an essential complement to pharmacological and psychotherapeutic treatment.

Table 37. Nutrients with neuroprotective and mood-modulating effect in bipolar disorder

Nutritious	Main source	Therapeutic effect
Omega-3 (EPA/DHA)	Oily fish, nuts	Anti-inflammatory, mood stabilizer
Magnesium	Spinach, almonds, avocado	Improves sleep and anxiety
Zinc and selenium	Seeds, shellfish	Support dopaminergic function
Vitamin D	Sun, fortified dairy	Regulates serotonin and immune system
Tryptophan	Turkey, oatmeal, banana	Natural precursor of serotonin
Polyphenols	Red fruits, green tea, cocoa	Antioxidant and neuroprotective

Every food can be a biochemical message that calms or alters the mind.

42.5 The Inflammatory Model of Bipolar Disorder

The connection between metabolism and inflammation explains why many patients develop insulin resistance, obesity, or metabolic syndrome, especially when using mood stabilizers or antipsychotics.

Inflammation affects the function of the blood-brain barrier, which increases emotional vulnerability.

Clinical recommendations:

- Control glucose, lipids and inflammatory markers.
- Introduce Mediterranean anti-inflammatory diet.
- Encourage intermittent fasting under medical supervision.
- Avoid excessive consumption of alcohol and refined sugars.

Inflammation is the silent fire that clutters the mind.

42.6 Integration with the DNP-21-B

Table 38 relates the different neurochemical profiles of the DNP-21-B model with frequent metabolic alterations and specific nutritional recommendations, highlighting the role of diet as a tool to modulate mood, stress, and neurobiological stability in bipolar disorder.

DNP-21-B makes it possible to associate certain neurochemical imbalances with the most appropriate diet for each profile.

Table 38. DNP-21-B profiles, associated metabolic alterations and nutritional recommendations

DNP-21-B Profile	Common metabolic disturbance	Nutritional recommendation
High dopamine	Anxiety, insomnia	Reduce caffeine and sugars
Low serotonin	Sadness, anhedonia	Increase tryptophan and omega-3
GABA Deficiency	Stress and irritability	Increase magnesium and fermented foods
Glutamate excess	Mental hyperactivity	Avoid monosodium glutamate and ultra-processed foods

Diet can modulate neurotransmitters in the same way as drugs, but without side effects.

42.7 Eating as a Therapeutic Act

Mindful eating is a daily form of preventive psychiatry. Every meal can be a dose of stability or a spark of imbalance. When the bipolar patient learns to nourish himself from biology and compassion, his body becomes a therapeutic ally. Eating well is an act of neurochemical love for oneself.

CHAPTER 43
Restful Sleep as a Cornerstone of Treatment

To sleep well is to stabilize the soul.

43.1 Sleep as a Neurochemical Regulator

In bipolar disorder, sleep is not a luxury, but a therapeutic mainstay. Sleep loss or dysregulation is one of the most sensitive and predictive symptoms of a relapse, both manic and depressive. In fact, up to 70% of manic episodes begin after several days of insomnia or reduced sleep.

Every restless night is a synapse that weakens. Getting adequate sleep not only recovers energy: it restores neurotransmitter balance, regulates the hypothalamic-pituitary-adrenal axis, and protects emotional stability.

43.2 Neurobiology of Sleep in the Bipolar Brain

Sleep is a choreography between melatonin, serotonin, GABA and glutamate. In patients with bipolarity, these systems usually present desynchronization of the circadian rhythm and alteration of the light-dark axis.

Mechanisms involved:

- Decreased melatonin: delays the onset of sleep and alters REM architecture.
- Excess nocturnal dopamine: causes mental hyperactivity.
- GABA deficiency: prevents physiological relaxation.
- Glutamate disruption: keeps the brain "on", even during rest.

The bipolar mind does not always sleep; Sometimes, just the light goes out.

43.3 Most Common Types of Sleep Disturbances

Table 39 describes the main types of sleep disturbances observed in bipolar disorder and their association with the different clinical phases, highlighting sleep as an early marker of affective destabilization and a priority therapeutic objective.

Table 39. Sleep Disorders and Associated Clinical Phases in Bipolar Disorder

Type of disorder	Features	Most common phase
Initial insomnia	Difficulty falling asleep	Mania or anxiety
Night awakenings	Fragmented sleep	Depression or stress
Short sleep without tiredness	Feeling of excessive energy	Hypomania
Hyperpersonmy	Oversleeping without real rest	Depressive phase
Inverted circadian rhythm	Nighttime activity and daytime sleepiness	Mixed States

43.4 Sleep Deprivation as a Trigger for Relapse

Studies show that even a single night of total deprivation can induce manic symptoms in vulnerable individuals. Chronic insomnia also raises cortisol and generates brain inflammation, which aggravates the risk of relapse.

Factors that perpetuate sleep deprivation:

- Psychological stress and racing thoughts.
- Caffeine, alcohol, or nicotine use.
- Nighttime use of screens (blue light).
- Irregular routines or night work.

Poor sleep is not just a symptom: it is a trigger.

43.5 Clinical Strategies for Restoring Sleep

a. Behavioral interventions:

- Maintain a fixed sleep and wake schedule.
- Avoid screens at least 60 minutes before bedtime.
- Reduce stimulant consumption.
- Associate the bed only with rest (not work or argument).
- Practice relaxation or deep breathing..

b. Pharmacological interventions:

- Melatonin or ramelteon: regulate circadian rhythm.
- Quetiapine or lurasidone: improve sleep without inducing addiction.
- Short-acting benzodiazepines: limited use in acute phases.
- Trazodone or mirtazapine: useful in depressive insomnia.

c. Complementary approaches:

- Mindfulness and yoga nidra: induce parasympathetic relaxation.
- Daylight therapy: stabilizes circadian rhythms.
- Supplements such as magnesium or theanine: promote neurological calm.

Sleeping well is a neurochemical recipe, not just a habit (Figure 42).

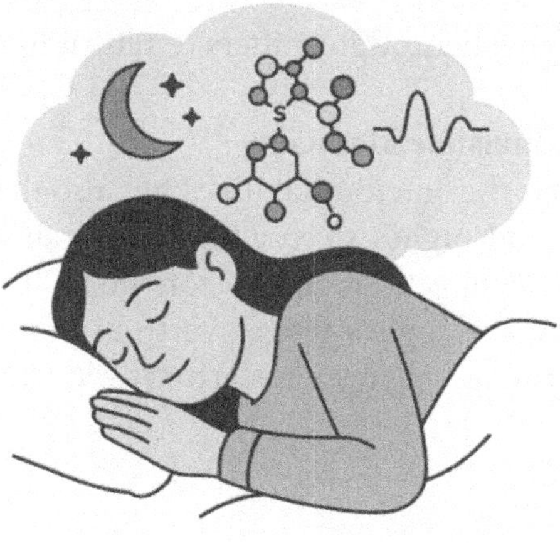

Figure 42. Restful sleep as a pillar of treatment in bipolar disorder. Light waves symbolize neurochemical restoration, circadian balance, and emotional serenity that emerge after deep rest.

43.6 Integration with the DNP-21-B Model

Table 40 relates the different neurochemical profiles of the DNP-21-B model with the most frequent sleep disturbances and suggested interventions. The approach to sleep is highlighted as a fundamental therapeutic axis for mood stability and the prevention of relapses in bipolar disorder. Sleep directly correlates with the neurochemical profiles described in DNP-21-B.

Table 40. DNP-21-B Profiles, Sleep Disturbances, and Intervention Strategies

DNP-21-B Profile	Typical sleep disturbance	Suggested Intervention
High dopamine	Insomnia, nocturnal euphoria	Fixed routine, melatonin, yoga
Low serotonin	Shallow sleep	Daytime exercise, tryptophan
GABA deficiency	Frequent awakenings	Relaxation techniques, GABAergic supplements
Glutamate excess	Nightmares, mental hyperactivity	Avoid screens, mindfulness, stabilizers

Sleep is allowing neurotransmitters to return to your home.

43.7 Rest as an Invisible Medicine

Restful sleep is the quietest stabilizer, but also the most powerful. Getting a good night's sleep allows the brain to reorganize emotions, repair connections, and restore hope. In the treatment of bipolar disorder, a night's rest is worth as much as a dose of lithium. Sleep is not giving up: it is starting over with a calm mind.

CHAPTER 44
Spirituality, Meaning of Life and Existential Crises

The soul also seeks chemical balance.

44.1 Beyond the Diagnosis: the Hunger for Meaning

The treatment of bipolar disorder cannot be limited to the biological. Although medication stabilizes mood, the meaning of life stabilizes identity.

In moments of crisis, many patients express questions that transcend psychiatry: "Why is this happening to me?", "What is the purpose of my existence?", "Am I something more than my ups and downs?". It is not only about balancing neurotransmitters, but about reconciling the mind with the soul.

Spirituality —understood not as religion, but as an inner search for coherence, hope and connection— has become a recognized protective factor in mental health (Figure 43).

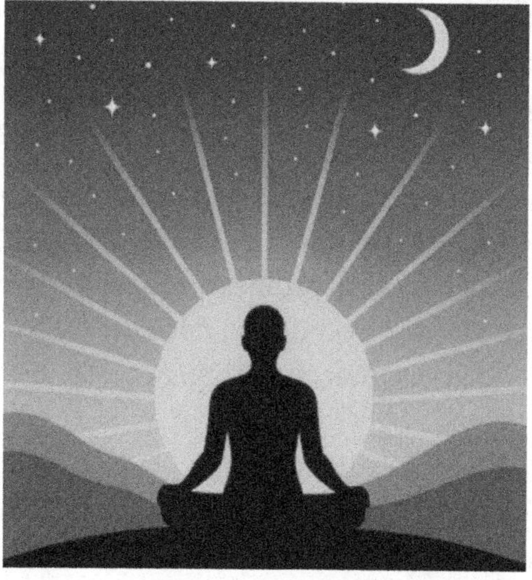

Figure 43. Conceptual representation of spirituality and the meaning of life in bipolar disorder. The inner light symbolizes the search for transcendence, the harmony between mind and soul, and the healing process that goes beyond the biological.

44.2 Neurobiology of Spirituality

Spirituality has an observable brain base. Neuroimaging studies show activation of the medial prefrontal section, the anterior cingulate and the inferior parietal lobe, regions associated with empathy, introspection and the perception of transcendence.

Identified neurochemical effects:

- Increased serotonin and oxytocin, linked to calmness and connection.
- Dopamine regulation, reducing impulsivity and euphoria.
- Activation of the vagus nerve, which induces states of deep relaxation.

Faith, meditation, or art can be as neurochemical as a dose of lithium.

44.3 Existential Crisis: when the Soul also Enters a Mixed Phase

During depressive phases, the bipolar patient may experience a deep spiritual emptiness: the feeling of loss of purpose, disconnection, or even "breakdown of the self". In manic phases, that same search can become euphoric or messianic, leading to delusional interpretations of reality.

Clinical example:

An artist with bipolar disorder describes that, in his manic phase, he "felt like he was chosen to save the world". After stabilization, he understood that this sensation was a distortion of the human desire for transcendence, not a divine vocation. Every spiritual crisis deserves understanding, not ridicule.

44.4 Spirituality and Resilience

Studies show that regular spiritual practice —be it meditation, prayer, contemplation, or contact with nature— decreases the recurrence of depressive episodes and improves adherence to treatment.

Psychological benefits:

- It increases hope and self-compassion.
- Strengthens sense of purpose and belonging.
- It reduces the fear of death and hopelessness.
- It promotes resilience in the face of guilt or stigma.

Spirituality does not replace medication, but it gives it meaning.

44.5 Clinical Integration of the Spiritual Approach

The psychiatrist or therapist can accompany the patient in this dimension without imposing beliefs. The goal is to reconnect the inner experience with the life narrative.

Helpful Clinical Tools:

- To explore the personal sense of faith, art or transcendence.
- Include in the interview this question: "What gives you strength to continue?"
- Recommend exercises of gratitude or daily contemplation.
- Encourage practices of service or community connection.

Therapeutic exercise:

The patient writes a letter addressed to his "future self", describing what it would mean for him to have overcome the pain. This symbolic act reinforces self-efficacy and hope.

44.6 Integration with the DNP-21-B

Table 41 explores the relationship between the neurochemical profiles of the DNP-21-B model and the different manifestations of spiritual experience, proposing therapeutic strategies that integrate contemplative, artistic, and community practices as a complement to the clinical approach, without contrasting spirituality and science. Spirituality also correlates with neurochemical balance.

Table 42. Spiritual dimension and neurochemical balance according to the DNP-21-B profile

DNP-21-B Profile	Associated spiritual dimension	Therapeutic strategy
High dopamine	Euphoria, spiritual grandeur	Guided Meditation & Grounding
Low serotonin	Hopelessness and existential emptiness	Gratitude and Art Practices
GABA deficiency	Spiritual anxiety or guilt	Mindful Breathing and Calm Prayer
High oxytocin	Interpersonal connection and compassion	Community activities and volunteering

Spirituality is not opposed to science: it complements it by reminding us why healing is worth it.

44.7 When the Mind Finds Its Purpose

Inner balance is not achieved only by correcting neurotransmitters, but by reconciling the body, mind and soul. Finding meaning in one's own existence transforms illness into a journey, pain into learning, and relapse into an opportunity to wake up. Mental health is not just emotional stability: it is feeling that life has meaning, even when it hurts.

CAPÍTULO 45
The Model of Medical Aikido Applied to Bipolarity (2A + 2B + 2C + 2D)

From the neurochemical storm to emotional mastery.

45.1 General Framework: Why "Aikido" in Mental Health?

Aikido does not seek to defeat an opponent, but to redirect his energy until he neutralizes the conflict without destroying. In bipolarity, the "force that arrives" is internal: surges of dopamine, glutamate and noradrenaline that push towards hypomania/mania or deficits in serotonin and GABA that drag depression and anxiety. Medical aikido proposes to recognize this biological inertia, to come into contact with it and to turn it into useful movement. It does not eliminate energy: it conducts it.

Central idea: every crisis contains information. If the patient learns to read it and move with it, he or she goes from "putting out fires" to practicing a discipline of daily self-regulation, with language, breathing, body, environment and treatment working in synchronization.

45.2 Practical Neurobiology of the Model

Each phase of the 2A + 2B + 2C + 2D medical aikido model (Anticipate, Analyze, Welcome, Benevolence, Control, Change, Tear Down and Dissolve) corresponds to a predominant brain circuit and a clinical lever.

Table 42 integrates the eight phases of the medical aikido model with their main neurobiological circuits and the corresponding regulatory levers. This provides a clinical framework that connects neuroscience, emotional regulation, and active therapeutic strategies for the management of bipolar disorder and other states of affective dysregulation.

Table 42. Medical Aikido Model (2A + 2B + 2C + 2D): Neurobiological Correlates and Therapeutic Levers

Phase	Circuit/Related	Regulating Lever
Anticipate	Salience network (insula–anterior cingulate) detects changes; noradrenaline ↑	Continuous monitoring, daily, wearables, prodromal signal detection
Analyze	Dorsolateral prefrontal cortex; mesocortical dopamine	Cognitive Reframing, Trigger Analysis, Micro-Adjustment Decisions
Welcome	Default network integrated with medial prefrontal cortex; serotonin	Acceptance without fusion, emotional labeling, brief interoceptive exposure
Benevolence	Affiliation system (oxytocin, orbitofrontal cortex)	Guided self-compassion, prosodic tone, confident touch
Control	GABAergic circuits; thalamus–bark	Diaphragmatic breathing, sensorimotor pauses, stimulus hygiene
Change	Glutamate/BDNF-dependent flexibility	Behavioral substitution, creative channel, micro-goals with feedback
Tear down	Executive network; Tonsillar extinction	Dispute of core beliefs, behavioral experiments
Dissolve	Endocannabinoids (anandamide), vagotonia	Release rumination, closing practice, rest rituals

Operational translation: each phase is not a slogan; It is a neurophysiological switch that the patient learns to press with specific and measurable techniques.

45.3 The 2A with Measurable Protocols

45.3.1 Anticipating: Signal Map and Risk Window

Objective: to detect changes ≥72 hours before overflow.

Tools:

- 3-column diary (morning/afternoon/evening) with 0–10 for energy, irritability, speed of thought, hours of actual sleep (actigraph or clock), caffeine/alcohol consumption, and conflict.
- Routine microbiomarkers: gut regularity, appetite, sugar/salt cravings (peripheral indicators of dopamine/serotonin).
- Personal prodromal signals (top-5 list). Frequent examples: reducing sleep without tiredness, more jokes and simultaneous projects, repeated "small" expenses, need to talk or in depression: starting to cancel plans, excessive use of bed/cell phone and hypersensitivity to rejection.

Activation thresholds:

- Hypomania/mania: sleep <5.5 h for 2 nights or <6.5 h for 3 nights, energy ≥7/10, unusual increased sociability.
- Depression: anhedonia ≥6/10 for 3 days, psychomotor slowness observed by third parties, nocturnal rumination >30 min.

Action Plan Level 1 (Yellow Traffic Light):

- Message to "observation partner" or designated family member: "I am on pre-alert, today I prioritize sleep, hydration, zero arguments".
- Behavioral readjustment: turn off screens 90 min before bedtime, remove caffeine after 2:00 p.m., simple dinner with tryptophan and magnesium, walk 20–30 min without stimulating music.
- Agreed medical link: if the signal persists for 72 hours, notify the psychiatrist for pharmacological microadjustment.

45.3.2 Analyze: Trigger Matrix and Microadjustment Decisions

Apply matrix 3×3 (biological-psychological-social × acute-subacute-chronic):

Real example: Carlos (33, bipolar I). Biological subacute trigger: two weeks of partial insomnia in shifts; psychological: new project with overdemand; Social: increase in departures. Decision: sleeps 9 hours two nights with the support of agreed medication, informs her boss to postpone deliveries, reduces social interaction by 5 days, resumes hydration and moderate exercise. Result: YMRS rises 4 points and returns to its baseline in a crisis-free week.

Clinical rule: do not make vital or financial decisions with sleep <6.5 h or mood >7/10 or <3/10.

45.4 The 2B with Guided Exercises

45.4.1 Welcome: 90-second Interoceptive Exposure

Instruction: When the wave appears (anger, euphoria, sadness) close your eyes for 90 seconds and describe precisely where you feel (chest, throat, forehead), temperature, texture, movement. Name: "this is energy X". No judgment. 4-4-6 breathing (inhale 4, hold 4, exhale 6). The 90-second rule reduces tonsillar reactivity and allows the cortex to retrieve speech.

Short script for the reader:

- "I feel pressure in my chest, hot, pulsating. I'm not the-pressure, I observe it. I inhale 4, hold 4, exhale 6. I can wait 90 seconds. I don't need to answer now".

45.4.2 Benevolence: Micro-self-compassion with Prosody

Self-criticism raises cortisol; Self-compassion done well raises oxytocin and lowers hyperarousal. Technique in 3 lines, in moderately low and slow voice (calming prosody):

1. Validation: "This hurts and it's difficult".
2. Shared humanity: "It happens to others too; I'm not alone".
3. Direction: "Today I treat myself like someone I care about: a small, kind step".

Real example: Lucía, 40 years old and with bipolar II disorder, used this triad before demanding meetings; it decreased their avoidance, increased their assertiveness, and reduced guilt-related relapses.

45.5 The 2C with Power Transfer Tools

45.5.1 Control: 6-stop Kit of 60-120 Seconds

- 4-7-8 breathing (3 repetitions) when the mind "runs".
- Hand on sternum + gentle pressure 30 s (stimulates lazy).
- Facial immersion in cold water 10-15 s or cold-splash to abort vegetative peaks.
- Grounding 5-4-3-2-1 (5 things you see, 4 things you touch...).
- Pencil and paper: list 3 concrete and feasible micro-actions (≤10 min each).
- Pause contract: "I stop the conversation if my volume exceeds 6/10".

Environmental Control Checklist:

- Warm light at night, blue filters, room ≤19 °C, sleep/sex only bed.
- Dose dopaminergic stimuli: music with moderate BPM, avoid night scrolling, soft white noise if there is hypervigilance.

45.5.2 Change: Behavioral Substitution and Creative Channel

Substitution rule: every impulsive behavior has a safe equivalent with the same "energetic charge".

- Expenses → "idea cart": write down and buy only 48-72 hours later if it still makes sense.
- Verbiage → "writing notebook": writing for 10 minutes without a filter, sharing only after reviewing it the next day.
- Sexual risk → "planned safe touch": emotional intimacy, vigorous exercise and cold shower, and then open conversation.

Case study: Roberto redirected the hypomania to “creative sprints” of 20 minutes of timed + 5 minutes of pause, 5 cycles/day, with a limit of screens at 8:30 p.m. He published his first photobook in 6 months, with stable sleep.

45.6 The 2D with Science of Thought and Closure

45.6.1 Tear Down: Belief Therapy with Behavioral Experiments

Frequent beliefs and suggested experiment:

- “Without mania I am not creative”.

Experiment: week of “stable creativity” with 25 min blocks, no intense music or caffeine late; measure creative output (pages, sketches). Many patients report superior quality with less mental noise.

- “If I stop, I get depressed”.

Experiment: introduce controlled naps of 20 min + gentle walking; register affection. It is proven that “stopping” is not equivalent to falling, but to recovering.

- “I'm a problem for my family”.

Experiment: request for concrete help of 10 min/day and subsequent feedback. The value of the patient in the system is clarified.

- “Internal court” technique.

Experiment: write automatic indictment, evidence for/against, reasonable verdict, and alternative conduct.

45.6.2 Dissolving: Neurobiological Closure Practices

- Writing 6 minutes before going to sleep (rumination discharge), tearing the paper or storing it in a “tomorrow I'll review it” envelope.
- Temperature ritual: warm shower 5 min followed by slightly cooler water 30 s; it induces a drop in core temperature and sleep.
- Short prayer/meditation or gratitude for 3 things; It raises oxytocin and changes mental framework.

- "Falling tide" visualization: as you exhale, imagine that the wave is receding.

Real case: Elena performed a monthly ritual of "reconciliation with the diagnosis": letter to her 20 years old self, 10 minutes of breathing, slow walk. Their embarrassment reactions decreased and adherence to lithium increased.

45.7 Differential Protocols by Phase

45.7.1 Hypomania/Mania Protocol (24-72 h)

1. Priority sleep: goal 8-9 h the first two nights. Melatonin 3-5 mg in the evening if indicated; Temporary negotiation of responsibilities.
2. Minimal stimulus: zero caffeine/energizers, soft music, avoid shopping/nightlife.
3. 4-7-8 breathing at the onset of euphoria or irritability; 3 series morning, afternoon, night.
4. Traffic light communication with family: "I'm on yellow, I need X". Avoid debates, money decisions, and impulsive posts.
5. Contact with a psychiatrist for microadjustment: atypical antipsychotic for rescue or stabilizer optimization according to the agreed plan.
6. Measured movement: gentle walk 20-30 min; avoid HIIT.
7. Measurement: YMRS/ASRM fast daily; to drop ≥6 points in 72 h as a target.

45.7.2 Bipolar Depression Protocol (7-14 days)

1. Graded behavioral activation: 3 blocks of 10-15 min/day at baseline (hygiene, sunlight, simple housework), work your way up to 5 blocks in a week.
2. Circadian rhythm: morning light 15-30 min, meals at fixed times, bed as a last resort during the day.
3. Planned micro-pleasure: harmless sensory activities (hot shower, tea, moderate nostalgic music) and brief human contact.

4. Language of benevolence: 90-second daily script in front of the mirror with the triad.
5. Safety monitor: suicidal ideation checked with traffic light (green/yellow/red) and visible safety plan.
6. Measurement: PHQ-9 or QIDS-SR weekly; Decline goal ≥5 points in 2–4 weeks along with medical adjustments.

45.8 DNP-21-B Integration: Custom Prescribing

Table 43 translates the predominant neurochemical profiles of the DNP-21-B model into frequent clinical risks and therapeutic microprescriptions based on the medical aikido model, offering brief, specific and easily applicable interventions for daily self-regulation and the prevention of affective decompensation.

Table 43. Therapeutic microprescription of medical aikido according to DNP-21-B profile

Dominant DNP-21-B Profile	Typical Risk	Aikido Microprescription
High dopamine	Impulsivity, spending, verbiage	Control: 4-7-8, turn off screens 90 min before, "idea cart 72 h"
Low serotonin	Pessimism, rumination	Benevolence + gratitude, sun exposure mornings, tryptophan/omega-3 foods
GABA deficiency	Somatic anxiety, insomnia	Diaphragmatic breathing, weight/deep stimulation, restorative yoga
Glutamate excess	Mixed states, hyperalert	Stimulus reduction, slow music, sensory breaks, avoiding MSG/ultra-processed
Low oxytocin	Insulation	Co-regulation: safe contact 20 s, psychoeducational groups, shared tasks

45.9 Working with Family and Couple: Relational Aikido

3-clause contracts:

1. Shared signal: Keyword for "pause" without discussion.
2. Yellow/red no-decision rule.
3. Positive feedback: recognizing a micro-achievement of the other every day.

Script when the tension rises:

1. Partner: "I'm noticing your faster voice and little sleep; I love you and it worries me. I propose a 10-minute pause and breathing together".
2. Patient: "Thank you for telling me like this. I take the pause; then we resumed".

45.10 Weekly Practice Plan (30 days, renewable)

Monday to Friday:

Morning: natural light 15-20 min; 5 minutes of breathing + check-in form (sleep, energy, purpose of the day); 25 min productive block.

Noon: 15-20 min walk; food with protein and fiber; check "idea cart".

Afternoon: two blocks of 25 minutes with a 5-minute break; grounding 5-4-3-2-1.

Night: 6 min written download; closing ritual (warm water + 90 s breathing); screens outside 90 min; light reading.

Saturday:

Week in Review: Sleep, Energy, and Events Chart. Identify what remained stable. Meaningful activity (nature/art).

Sunday:

Gentle planning: micro-goals, meals, rest, a social commitment. Close with gratitude.

45.11 Measurement-Based Care

- Baseline and follow-up: YMRS/ASRM for hypomania/mania, PHQ-9 or QIDS-SR for depression, Insomnia Severity Index if applicable.

- Process indicators: hours of sleep, "yellow days", number of pauses applied, adherence to breathing and night closure.
- Outcome indicators: ↓ hospitalizations/emergencies, ↓ family conflicts, ↑ functional days, ↑ self-efficacy.

45.12 Motivating Ending Vignettes

Ana (teacher, bipolar II) turned her monthly "black week" into an "intensive care week": she reduced her schedule by 30%, increased sleep and sensory micropleasures, and maintained three daily micro-productivitys. Two semesters without medical leave.

Mario (entrepreneur, bipolar I) feared losing his creative spark as he stabilized. With the Change phase, he designed a "study of ideas" with time limits and mandatory rest. He billed more with less chaos and improved his relationship.

Claudia (resident physician) learned welcome and control with cold water and breathing when she noticed impulsive nighttime spending. In 6 months, zero new debt and higher self-esteem (Figure 44).

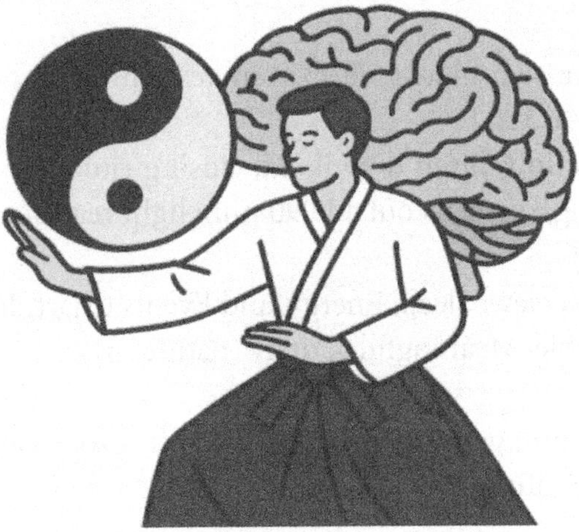

Figure 44. Conceptual representation of the model of medical aikido applied to bipolar disorder. The balance between the brain and the yin yang symbol reflects the redirection of emotional energy and the transformation of inner conflict into neurochemical harmony.

45.13 Transforming Practice

Medical aikido is not a pretty theory; It is a daily discipline that turns chemical waves into dance steps. Anticipate and analyze provide mapping; welcome and benevolence offer safe soil; control and change give direction; tearing down and dissolving open up space to live with dignity and purpose. Bipolarity ceases to be a war and becomes a dojo: a training place for the mind and heart.

PART IX.
Recovery and Resilience

CHAPTER 46
What Does This Remission Mean?

Remission is not the end of the road,
but the art of maintaining balance.

46.1 Remission Does not Mean Definitive Cure

In bipolar disorder, "remission" means that clinical symptoms subside to a subthreshold level and the patient regains sufficient neuroemotional stability to safely resume life. It does not imply a definitive cure or the permanent absence of relapses. Remission is a phase of stability that requires active surveillance, fine therapeutic adjustments, and regimented lifestyle habits to sustain itself over time.

46.2 Types of Remission: Clinical, Syndromic and Functional

Clinical remission: reduction of affective symptoms below established thresholds on validated scales (e.g., YMRS $\leq$ 4 for mania; MADRS or QIDS in minimum range; CGI-BP $\leq$ 2).

Syndromic remission: absence of complete diagnostic criteria for manic, hypomanic, or depressive episodes for a minimum period of time (usually $\geq$ 8 weeks).

Functional remission: recovery of functioning in work/school, relationships and self-care, measurable with scales such as FAST, WHO-DAS or the patient's previous level of performance. The clinical goal is not just to silence symptoms, but to restore roles and purpose.

46.3 Stabilization Does not Mean Cure

Stabilization describes a dynamic state maintained by treatment, habits, and psychosocial support. The physiology of bipolar vulnerability persists (circadian reactivity, dopaminergic/serotonergic lability, susceptibility to stress). Therefore, even in remission, there is a baseline risk of relapse if adherence decreases, sleep dysregulation is dysregulated or stressors appear. Thinking about "total cure" favors early abandonment of treatment and increases the risk of cycling.

46.4 Practical Criteria for Sustained Remission

- Stable subclinical symptoms for at least 8 to 12 weeks.
- Regular sleep 7-9 h, short latency, no prolonged awakenings, consistent chronotype.
- Consistent activity rhythms: predictable meal, work, and exercise times.
- Proper executive function: planning, sustained attention, impulse control.
- Self-injurious risk absent and judgment preserved. Proven pharmacological adherence and acceptable tolerability. Active support network and early signs plan implemented.

46.5 How Do We Measure Remission?: Minimum Follow-up Bacteria

- **Mood and energy:** YMRS for residual manic symptoms; PHQ-9, MADRS, or QIDS for residual depressive symptoms.
- **Anxiety and sleep:** GAD-7 and a 2-week sleep diary or actigraphy when possible.
- **Operation:** FAST or WHO-DAS every 1-3 months in the maintenance phase.
- **Brief cognition:** Timed tests of attention/processing speed (e.g., Symbol Digit Modality Test) when cognitive complaints are present.
- **Global severity:** CGI-BP and subjective self-assessment of well-being (0-10).

- **Biological-therapeutic:** plasma levels when appropriate (lithium, valproate), metabolic profile if antipsychotics are used, TSH if lithium is present, and hepatic/hematological parameters according to drugs

46.6 Summary Neurobiology of Remission

During remission, mesolimbic dopaminergic hyperreactivity decreases and prefrontal modulation is restored, while the circadian axis (suprachiasmatic nucleus) recovers synchrony with light-dark signals and routines. Vulnerabilities persist in cognitive control networks, salience, and limbic-prefrontal regulation, so the brain remains "sensitized" to stress, sleep deprivation, and dopaminergic/stimulant substances.

46.7 Residuals that Matter: Small Symptoms, Big Risks

- Minimal mixed symptoms (irritability, mild cognitive acceleration) increase the likelihood of swerving.
- Insomnia and sleep schedule variability predict manic relapse; hypersomnia and anerggia, depressive relapse.
- Subclinical anhedonia, fatigue, or bradypsychia are associated with poorer functioning and adherence.
- Microimpulsivity (shopping, reckless driving, hyperconnectivity in networks) can anticipate hypomanic decompensation.

46.8 Recommended Maintenance Duration After Referral

After a first episode: consider maintenance for at least 12-24 months, individualizing by family burden, severity and preferences.

After two or more episodes, severe, mixed or high-risk episodes: indefinite maintenance with periodic reviews of the benefit-risk balance.

If dose reductions are evaluated, they should be gradual and outside of higher-risk seasons, with an intensive monitoring plan.

46.9 Therapeutic Principles in Remission

- **Pharmacological:** maintain the effective stabilizer at the minimum effective dose; verify levels (lithium 0.6–0.8 mEq/L in typical maintenance), optimize the motrigine in depressive polarity, and minimize unnecessary polypharmacy. Evaluate depot antipsychotic if there were relapses due to adherence.
- **Specific psychotherapies:** Structured psychoeducation, interpersonal social rhythm therapy (IPSRT), focused family therapy (FFT), and bipolar-adapted CBT reduce relapse and improve functioning.
- **Rhythms and lifestyle:** fixed sleep schedule, exposure to morning light, regular aerobic exercise, eating with stable schedules, reducing alcohol and caffeine, avoiding stimulant substances.
- **Iatrogenic prevention:** caution with antidepressants in bipolar I and with a history of reversal; if used, with stabilizer and close monitoring.
- **Comorbidities:** treat anxiety, ADHD, substance use, and sleep disorders because they erode remission.

46.10 Early Signs and Rapid Action Plan

Define with the patient their personal markers: changes in sleep, speed of thought, spending, verbiage, irritability, withdrawal, hopelessness, ideas of guilt.

Assign action thresholds: for example, if there are 2 nights with < 6 h of sleep or GAD-7 goes up ≥ 5 points, activate plan.

Plan steps: immediate contact with the team, brief adjustment of medication according to pre-agreed schedule, reinforced sleep hygiene, reduction of demands and increase of family support.

Toolbox: diaphragmatic breathing, digital nighttime routine, exposure to morning light, list of "anchor activities" and temporary blocking of purchases in apps if there is an impulsive risk.

46.11 Brief Clinical Maintenance Algorithm

Confirm syndromic and functional remission → optimize base drug at the lowest effective dose and verify tolerability → select needs-based psychotherapy → establish circadian routine with objective metrics → create early signs plan and agree on microadjustments allowed → schedule quarterly monitoring (or monthly if high risk) with a standardized brief battery → review comorbidities and adherence at each visit → continuous education for patient and family.

46.12 Patient Education: How to Explain It in Consultation?

"Being in remission means that your brain has regained its balance and that your symptoms are 'under the radar'. It's not your fault if there's biological vulnerability, but it's your responsibility — and ours— to maintain sleep rhythms, medication, and an early signs plan. This way we reduce the risk of relapse and help you build a full life".

46.13 Referral Checklist for the control Visit

- Stable subclinical symptoms ≥ 8 weeks.
- Regular sleep without prolonged awakenings.
- FAST/Operating within Expected Range.
- 90% ≥ adhesion verified.
- Tolerable adverse effects and up-to-date laboratories.
- Early signs plan reviewed with family.
- Life goals and significant activities in progress.

46.14 Weekly Self-Monitoring Sheet (Suggested Format)

- Sleep: bedtime/wake-up, total hours, naps, quality 0-10.
  Mood and energy: scale 0-10.
- Impulsivity/anxiety: scale 0-10 and concrete examples.
- Routines: exercise, meals on schedule, exposure to morning light.

- Adherence: omissions of dose and reason.
- Stress events: what happened and how was it managed?
- Actions taken: regulation techniques, contact with equipment, permitted settings.

46.15 Conclusion

Remission is a clinical achievement and a life project. It is sustained by science, habits, and community. Stabilization is not the ultimate cure, but it is the platform from which patients can study, work, love, and create safely (Figure 45).

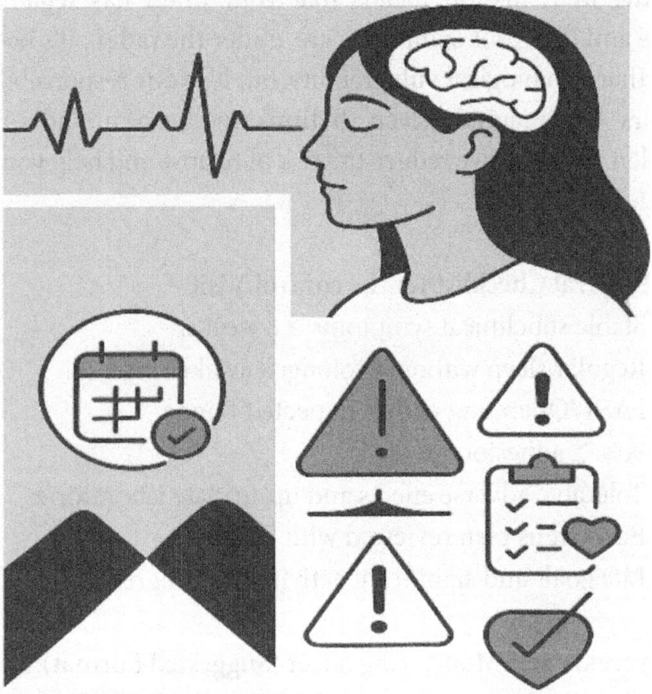

Figure 45. Remission in bipolar disorder represents a phase of clinical stability with subthreshold symptoms, but with a risk of relapse if continuous monitoring and healthy habits are not maintained.

CHAPTER 47
Life Projects with Bipolarity: Realism and Hope

Living with bipolarity is not giving up dreaming,
but learning to dream with our feet in biology.

47.1 Lucid Stability: the Alchemy between Biology and Purpose

To live with bipolar disorder is to learn to negotiate with the most powerful energy in the human mind: the oscillation between expansion and contraction. Those who have gone through mania and depression know the peak of excess and the abyss of emptiness. But between the two extremes there is a third way: lucid stability, where the individual does not renounce his passion, but domesticates it, channels it and turns it into a life project. In this alchemy between biology and purpose, true recovery is built.

Modern science no longer defines remission only as the absence of symptoms, but as the restoration of functionality, identity, and meaning in life. The question is not "Am I cured?" but "How can I live fully within my biology?" This chapter explores that answer from neuroscience, clinical psychology, and human experience.

47.2 Therapeutic Realism: the Wisdom of the Midpoint

Every bipolar person moves between two illusions: denial ("I don't need medication anymore") and fatalism ("I will never be able to be happy"). Therapeutic realism is the emotional maturity that is reached when the patient understands that vulnerability does not eliminate freedom, but conditions and guides it.

This balance requires a process of neurobiological insight: understanding that the disorder is not just a psychological label, but a pattern of hyperconnectivity between limbic networks (amygdala, insula) and dysfunction in prefrontal control networks (dorsolateral, orbitofrontal). In remission, these networks are retrained through routine, sleep and pharmacological adherence, allowing brain stability that makes it possible to design long-term goals. Therapeutic realism means accepting that the brain has cycles, but consciousness can learn to navigate them.

47.3 Redefining Success: from the Heroic Ideal to the Life Process

In the classic model of success, we are taught to accumulate external achievements. In the bipolar mind model, success should be measured in terms of internal coherence, functional continuity, and self-acceptance. Success is not "not having relapses", but coming back with more wisdom every time you fall. In neuropsychology, this is associated with apt plasticity: the brain's ability to reorganize itself after affective episodes and develop new coping strategies.

Functional neuroimaging studies show that patients who achieve prolonged stability have greater connectivity between the ventromedial prefrontal cortex and the hippocampus, areas that are involved in emotion regulation and autobiographical integration. In other words, remembering without reliving, learning without blaming oneself, rebuilding oneself without idealizing perfection.

47.4 Axes of the Stable Life Project

A sustainable life project requires synchronizing three systems: biological, psychological and existential.

1. **Biological axis. Rhythm and energy:**

The bipolar brain is a sensitive clock. Small disturbances in sleep or schedules can desynchronize the suprachiasmatic nucleus and alter the release of dopamine, melatonin, and cortisol. Therefore, circadian stability is not advice: it is a medical prescription. Sleeping, eating, and exposing yourself to sunlight at regular times acts as a natural chronobiological therapy.

2. **Psychological axes. Self-regulation and Purpose:**

Psychotherapy must transcend symptomatic relief. The most effective therapies are those that link the patient's identity with their life purpose. Interpersonal social rhythm therapy (IPSRT) and acceptance and commitment therapy (ACT) have been shown to increase adherence, decrease relapse, and reinforce self-compassion. The goal is not to eliminate episodes, but to teach the patient to read their own emotional barometer.

3. **Existential axis. Meaning and significance:**

People with bipolar disorder often have a high aesthetic and moral sensitivity. Channeling that intensity into art, spirituality, or social service transforms hypersensitivity into a source of meaning. Viktor Frankl put it precisely: "Whoever has a reason to live can endure almost any how".

47.5 Neurobiology of Hope

Hope is a complex neurochemical experience. In remission, the balance between dopamine (motivation), serotonin (satisfaction), and GABA (tranquility) allows for a sense of purpose without overstimulation.

The anterior cingulate cortex and the mesocorticolimbic system participate in the representation of future goals. When these circuits are synchronized, the mind can project itself forward without falling into the dopaminergic excess of mania or the serotonergic inhibition of depression.

Functional resonance studies (Kringelbach et al., 2021) demonstrate that gratitude practice and realistic planning simultaneously activate the ventral striatum (reward center) and medial prefrontal cortex (regulation center), generating a stable sense of active, not illusory, hope.

47.6 Therapies of Meaning and Reinvention

The most advanced psychotherapeutic treatment for the bipolar remission stage combines techniques from:

- Structured psychoeducation.
- Bipolar-adapted cognitive therapy (CBT-BP).
- Neuroregulatory mindfulness.
- Value therapy and logotherapy.

The therapist is not a "crisis controller", but an architect of meaning. It accompanies the patient to reconstruct their life narrative, integrating the episodes as learning chapters, not as identity fractures.

47.7 Clinical Example

Javier, 42, a musician and university professor, experienced three serious manic episodes and prolonged depression. After his stabilization with lithium and lamotrigine, he adopted a strict sleep routine and reduced his caffeine intake.

In therapy, she discovered that her creativity did not depend on mania, but on discipline. He composed his most important work during a year of stability. Today she teaches young people with affective disorders, integrating music and emotional neuroeducation. His life project was not to abandon his art, but to redefine it from serenity.

47.8 Practical Strategies

- Personal circadian map: Record daily energy peaks and troughs to plan demanding cognitive tasks at times of greatest stability.
- Purpose therapeutic contract: define three realistic annual goals linked to personal values.
- Overflow prevention plan: written protocols for insomnia, irritability or incipient euphoria.
- Quarterly review of goals: in the medical-therapeutic team, not only evaluate symptoms, but also life satisfaction.

47.9 The Environment as a Regulatory System

Human relationships function as biological co-regulators. Research on "affective synchrony" shows that people close to the patient modulate their heart, hormonal, and emotional rhythms. That's why an empathetic and predictable environment can reduce the frequency of relapses. Educating the family, the couple and the work environment is a form of primary prevention.

47.10 From Ideal Sleep to Sustainable Purpose

Bipolar disorder does not destroy dreams: it purifies them. It forces us to replace overflowing ambition with sustainable purpose. It teaches that fulfillment is not about living at the top or avoiding the valley, but about building a stable bridge between the two.

Hope is no longer naïve and becomes a neuroemotional discipline: a daily training in coherence, awareness and meaning. That is the real clinical and human victory (Figure 46).

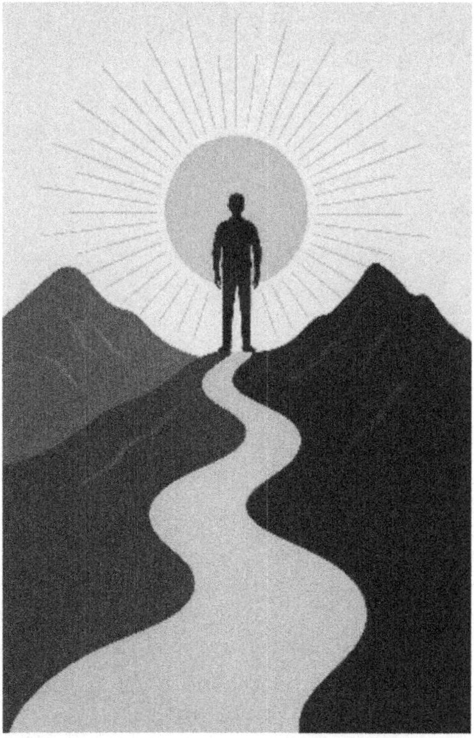

Figure 46. The golden path symbolizes the hope and vital direction of the bipolar patient who is moving towards the light of inner stability.

CHAPTER 48
Doctor-patient Relationship

Medication regulates the brain;
The therapeutic relationship sustains the person.

48.1 Enduring Therapeutic Alliance

In the treatment of bipolar disorder, medication stabilizes the brain, but the therapeutic alliance sustains life. A strong patient-doctor bond is the most consistent factor in long-term recovery, beyond drugs, crises, and changes in environment.

The bipolar patient, due to the very oscillating nature of his biology, needs a relationship that combines emotional stability, empathic authority and longitudinal accompaniment. This relationship is not vertical or paternalistic, but a pact of trust between two specialists: the doctor in neurochemistry, the patient in his own inner experience.

48.2 The neurobiology of the therapeutic link

The human brain is designed for relationship. The doctor-patient alliance activates neurobiological systems of trust, similar to those that operate in secure attachment bonds.

During the consultation, the release of oxytocin, activation of the orbitofrontal cortex, and modulation of the HPA (hypothalamic-pituitary-adrenal) axis reduce stress and facilitate adherence.

A calm voice, a congruent gaze, and the predictability of encounters have a measurable physiological effect: they lower cortisol, stabilize the heart rate, and reinforce the sense of subjective control.

The therapeutic relationship, in this context, is not sentimentality: it is interpersonal neuroregulation.

48.3 Phases of the Alliance in the Bipolar Patient

1. Initial containment phase: during diagnosis or acute crisis, the patient needs an anchor doctor. He is not looking for speeches, but for presence and clarity.
2. Collaboration phase: once stabilized, shared goals are established: relapse prevention, dose adjustment, sleep management and family education.
3. Supervised autonomy phase: the patient assumes co-responsibility and learns to self-monitor their symptoms. The goal is not dependence, but therapeutic maturity.
4. Reunion phase: after a relapse, the bond is reevaluated and renewed. The doctor avoids lawsuits; the patient learns that relapse is not failure, but part of the evolutionary process.

48.4 Clinical Empathy and Professional Boundaries

Empathy is a therapeutic modulator, but without limits it becomes risk. The professional must understand the emotion without absorbing it, contain it without merging, accompany without saving.

Studies in empathic neuroscience show that the activation of the right supramarginal gyrus allows the therapist to maintain cognitive compassion without affective contagion. In practice, this translates into deep listening, validating language, and protective emotional neutrality.

The balance between warmth and containment builds trust and mutual respect.

48.5 Effective Therapeutic Communication

- Clear, non-technical language: "Your medication helps your brain maintain its natural rhythm", is more helpful than "regulating dopaminergic neurotransmitters".
- Emotional validation: acknowledging suffering without exaggerating it. "I understand this is tough, but you're making progress".

- Shared education: use diagrams, calendars, or apps to track symptoms.
- Two-way feedback: the patient reports side effects; the doctor adapts without imposing.
- Therapeutic humor: a touch of respectful humor can ease tension and humanize the consultation.

48.6 Confidence, Adherence and Prognosis

The evidence is overwhelming: a strong therapeutic alliance predicts a better outcome than the simple choice of drug. Meta-analysis (De Fruyt et al., 2020; Miklowitz, 2022) show that patients who trust their psychiatrist have 30–50% fewer relapses and greater adherence to lithium or lamotrigine.

Trust is built on three pillars:

- Coherence: saying what you do and doing what you say.
- Competence: up-to-date knowledge and ability to explain.
- Continuity: avoid unnecessary rotations of professionals, since the longitudinal link acts as an emotional stabilizer.

48.7 The Doctor as a Regulating Mirror

The psychiatrist doesn't just prescribe:he models emotional regulation. When the patient is excited, the doctor's calm serves as an anchor; When depressed, his empathic tone works as a moderate stimulus.

The consultation becomes a "prefrontal MRI room", where the stability of the clinician facilitates the cortical reorganization of the patient. This explains why the doctor's relational style directly influences resilience circuits, enhancing positive neuroplasticity.

48.8 The Patient as the Protagonist

A lasting alliance does not infantilize. The patient must participate in decision-making, know the risks and benefits of each option, and learn to communicate their symptoms accurately.

The physician who fosters autonomy promotes an observant self, capable of recognizing mental states without being dominated by them. The dialogue goes from being hierarchical ("you obey") to co-creative ("we work together to take care of your mind").

48.9 Critical Moments: Rupture and Repair

Every therapeutic relationship goes through tensions: mistrust, adverse effects, differences in approach or mutual fatigue. The handling of these ruptures defines their maturity.

A doctor who can say: "I'm sorry if something I said made you feel judged, let's review how to continue better" transmits humanity without losing authority. Bond repair teaches the patient something essential: that relationships can survive conflict without destroying each other. This experience is therapeutic in itself.

48.10 The Future of the Alliance: Telemedicine and Digital Humanity

Virtuality offers continuity and access, but it should not replace emotional presence.

The screen can mediate the word, but it should not erase the gaze. The challenge of modern psychiatry is to combine technology with compassion. In the coming years, artificial intelligence, digital biomarkers and circadian monitoring may complement clinical judgment, but they will never replace the human trust that is born between two consciences that listen to each other.

48.11 Existential Alliance

In bipolar disorder, the doctor-patient relationship is more than a therapeutic contract: it is an existential alliance. The doctor learns from the patient's courage; the patient is sustained by the science and serenity of the doctor.

Together they form a neurohuman equation where stability is built in two directions: from the synapse to the soul, from the soul to the synapse. When trust becomes a method, psychiatry ceases to be just crisis medicine and becomes a medicine of hope (Figure 47).

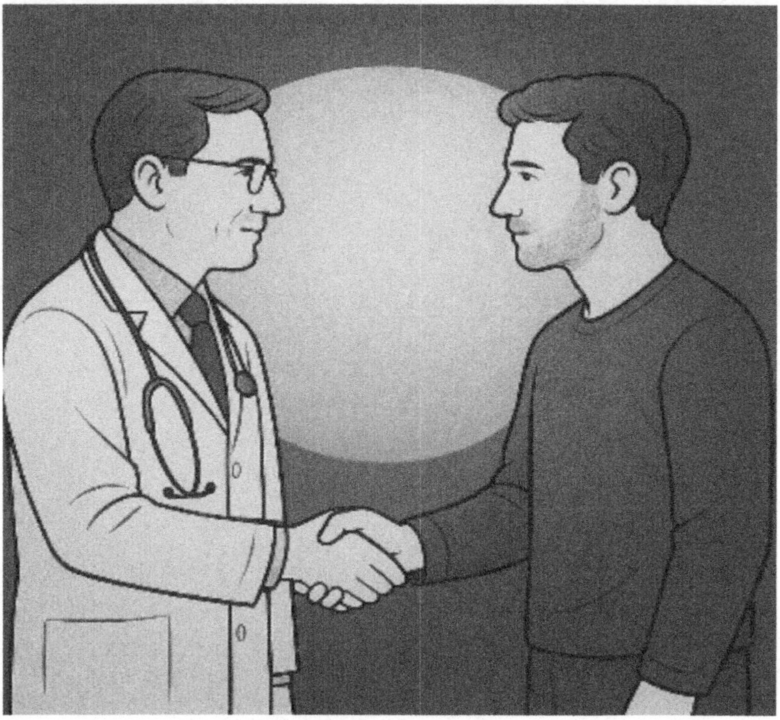

Figure 47. The therapeutic alliance: encounter between science and humanity, where trust becomes the most lasting medicine.

CHAPTER 49
Relapse Prevention: Early Signs and Action Plans

Before the crisis, the brain always sends signals.

49.1 Introduction

In bipolar disorder, preventing a relapse is not an act of luck, but a sustained neurobiological strategy. Relapse does not happen from one day to the next; It is announced in the subtle language of the body, sleep, energy, and mind.

Recognizing those cues before the episode sets in makes the difference between control and decompensation. The aim of this chapter is to transform surveillance into knowledge, fear into foresight, and vulnerability into power.

49.2 Understanding the Neurobiological Terrain of Risk

Bipolar relapse is associated with progressive dysregulation of the dopaminergic, serotonergic, and circadian systems.

- In mania, mesolimbic dopaminergic hypersensitivity is observed: the reward system is activated with minimal stimulation (lack of sleep, stress, stimulants).
- In depression there is serotonergic hypoactivity and functional hypofrontality, accompanied by a decrease in BDNF (brain neurotrophic factor), which reduces neuronal plasticity.
- Both extremes share a common denominator: desynchronization of the sleep-wake rhythm and loss of emotional homeostasis.

For this reason, the monitoring of circadian rhythms and sleep is one of the most sensitive markers to anticipate relapses.

49.3 The Three Phases of Relapse

1. Invisible prodrome (precursor) phase: minimal changes in energy, sleep, speed of thought, or irritability.
2. Amplification phase: Symptoms begin to affect behavior and relationships; the patient can still correct course if intervention is done early.
3. Phase of lack of control: the episode sets in, compromising judgment and functionality, requiring immediate medical intervention.

Effective therapeutic work occurs between the first and second phases, when there is still awareness and capacity for self-correction.

49.4 Specific Early Signs

Indicators of manic or hypomanic turn:

- Reduced sleep (<5 h for two nights in a row) without fatigue.
- Unusual increase in energy, productivity, or verbiage.
- Irritability, high mood, or sense of grandiosity.
- Impulsive spending, increased libido, or simultaneous multiple projects.
- Difficulty concentrating on routine tasks.
- Feeling "brighter, faster, or more capable than others".

Indicators of depressive relapse:

- Increased sleep or persistent insomnia.
- Disproportionate fatigue and anhedonia.
- Feeling of emptiness, guilt or worthlessness.
- Decreased social communication.
- Disinterest in medication or medical follow-up.
- Thoughts of hopelessness or self-destructive ideation.

Mixed (more dangerous) indicators:

- Extreme irritability with easy crying.
- High energy but depressed mood.

- Impulsivity with hopelessness.
- Mental acceleration with intense anxiety.

These states require immediate action, as they are the ones with the highest suicide risk.

49.5 The 10 Strongest Predictors of Relapse

1. Sleep deprivation or irregularity.
2. Suspension or poor adherence to treatment.
3. Consumption of alcohol, caffeine or stimulants.
4. Acute psychosocial stress (breakups, losses, work overload).
5. Seasonal changes (spring and autumn).
6. Jet lag or long trips.
7. Physical illness, fever, or infections.
8. Pregnancy or postpartum in women with a history of bipolar.
9. Previous history of mixed episodes or fast cyclers.
10. Lack of social support or therapeutic breaks.

49.6 Neuropsychoeducation: Teaching How to Read the Signs

Modern psychoeducation is not limited to teaching the diagnosis, but to training the mind to detect physiological and emotional micro-changes.

The patient must learn to observe:

- your sleep pattern (with actigraph or digital diary),
- your daily energy level (scale 1–10),
- your automatic thoughts,
- their connection habits (use of networks, verbal activity, spending, sexuality).

This self-observation turns the patient into their own biosensor, complementing the medical work.

49.7 Construction of the Personal Prevention Plan

An effective plan should be written, shared with the family and health team, and reviewed every three months. Includes:

A. My baseline:

- Average sleep schedule.
- Normal level of energy and concentration.
- Typical mood and communication style.

B. My Early Signs:

Each person has his or her "prodromal imprint". Some notice that they speak faster, others that they isolate themselves or that everything bothers them. Identifying those personal brands is key.

C. My immediate actions:

- Contact your doctor or therapist.
- Increase sleep hygiene (no screens, nighttime routine).
- Reduce caffeine, alcohol, and intense social activity.
- Resume medication or adjust the dose if it was stopped.
- Inform a trusted person for accompaniment.

D. My support networks:

Record emergency contacts, therapist, psychiatrist, key family members, and crisis lines.

49.8 The Role of the Environment

The functional environment as an external alarm system. The family or couple may notice changes before the patient himself. It's critical to create a common language: instead of "you're weird", say "I've noticed that you're sleeping less and talking faster, shall we review your plan together?" Empathy and precision avoid conflict and promote early intervention.

49.9 Technology and Prevention

Current advances make it possible to use smartwatches, sleep tracking apps, and circadian monitoring platforms to detect alterations in rhythm before the episode appears.

Recent studies (Hidalgo-Mazzei et al., 2023) show that digital monitoring reduces hospitalizations and improves adherence, especially when the patient has an active participation in the interpretation of their data.

49.10 Psychology of Prevention

Preventing a relapse isn't just a cognitive task; it requires retraining the mind to tolerate stability.

Some patients, unconsciously, feel more "alive" in hypomania and experience stability as boredom. That's why part of therapy involves redefining calm as a creative state and not an empty one. Lasting prevention combines self-knowledge, discipline and acceptance of one's own biological rhythm.

49.11 Psychiatric Emergencies and First Aid

If early signs progress despite measures, you should:

- Communicate to the doctor without delay.
- Suspend impulsive decisions (moving, breakups, investments).
- Avoid driving or handling finances if there is impaired judgment.
- Activate a crisis plan and face-to-face accompaniment.

The essential ethical principle: act at the first symptom, not the last.

49.12 Conclusions

The future of bipolar treatment lies not only in new drugs, but in the ability of each patient to become a lucid observer of his or her own mind.

Relapse prevention is the art of living in sync with oneself: recognizing the signs, acting without panic, and holding stability as a form of wisdom. Every stable day isn't just a medical achievement —it's a spiritual victory over chaos (Figure 48).

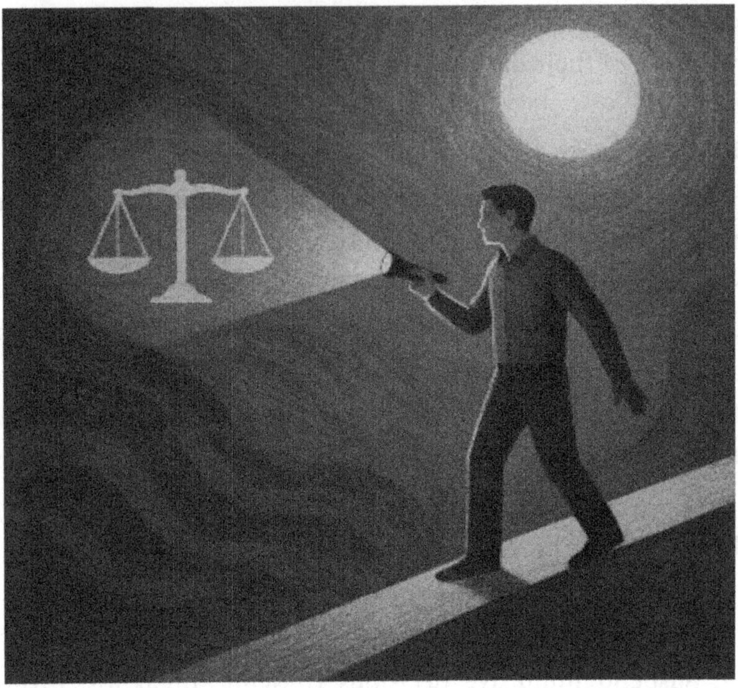

Figure 48. Active surveillance illuminates the signs of imbalance before the episode emerges. Prevention is a form of wisdom in motion.

CHAPTER 50
Recovery Stories: Patients Who Inspire

Recovery does not erase the past:
it transforms it into useful experience.

50.1 Introduction

Every bipolar recovery is a story of alchemy. The person transforms the raw material of suffering —chemical chaos, guilt, loss of control— into an architecture of stability and purpose. Medicine offers the blueprints, psychotherapy provides the tools, but the real reconstruction is done by the patient himself, day after day, molecule after molecule, thought after thought. Recovery is not a straight line or a spontaneous miracle: it is an emotional discipline that is renewed every morning.

Contemporary neuroscience has shown that the bipolar brain retains an extraordinary quality: plasticity. Connections that are once disorganized can be retrained, damaged synapses can be reinforced, and circuits that were once a source of instability can become pathways of resilience. Hope, when practiced methodically, is also a form of invisible neurosurgery.

In this chapter, we present real stories —transformed to preserve identity— that illustrate how science and will can build a new existence on the ruins of imbalance. They are human stories, but they are also clinical models of neuroadaptation, circadian balance and existential resignification.

50.2 Laura, the Architect of Rhythm

Civil engineer, 34 years old. For a decade he mistook hypomania for creativity and depression for failure. His mind oscillated like a pendulum between monumental projects and abysmal exhaustion. Hospitalization was his turning point. There he understood that stability was not boredom, but biological precision.

With the help of her psychiatrist and therapist, she designed a mathematical routine: always sleep at 11, get up at 7, eat at the same time, alternate work and rest, and go out every morning to receive sunlight. At first it was an imposition, then it became a ritual, finally an identity.

Today he runs a sustainable engineering company and teaches about mental health at international conferences. "Rhythm is my invisible architecture", he says. Their case shows how constancy modifies the connectivity between the suprachiasmatic nucleus and the prefrontal cortex: each respected schedule becomes a neurological brick that sustains stability.

50.3 Andrew, the Mentor of the Second Chance

Entrepreneur and creative, 47 years old. His manic episode led him to lose family, job and credibility. When he woke up from the euphoria, he fell into a devastating depression. Her recovery began when a therapist taught her the difference between guilt and responsibility. He learned that accepting does not mean justifying, and that forgiving oneself does not imply forgetting, but integrating.

She participated in cognitive therapy groups and mindfulness programs for self-compassion. In the process, he discovered that he could teach others what he had learned. Today she leads a mentoring organization for young people with affective disorders. He speaks with moral authority and serenity. "It's not about erasing the past, it's about building something worthy on top of it".

Studies in affective neuroscience show that self-compassion activates the anterior cingulate cortex and deactivates the self-attack circuit of the insula, which generates physiological relief that Andrés turned into a philosophy of life.

50.4 Diana, the Artist Who Painted Her Balance

A 28 years old painter and poet, diagnosed with mixed bipolar disorder. In his stages of crisis, his paintings were chaotic, full of explosive colors and overflowing strokes.

In therapy, her psychiatrist and psychologist decided to integrate art therapy and psychoeducation into a single process. He learned to recognize his emotional palette: reds for euphoria, grays for fatigue, blues for calm.

His canvas was transformed into a form of emotional self-regulation. Each brushstroke was a controlled release of dopamine. His Brain in Balance series was exhibited in museums and universities, and today he uses his art to educate other patients. "I used to paint to escape. Now I paint to understand".

Neuroimaging studies confirm that the creative act stimulates the orbitofrontal cortex, modulating the reward system and balancing the dopaminergic axis. Diana unknowingly turned art into a neurotherapeutic tool.

50.5 Samuel, the Body as Medicine

A 52 years old former athlete, he went through three hospitalizations and multiple relapses. No dose fully stabilized him until he understood that his body was part of the treatment. He began to apply a strategy based on neurophysiology: running every morning at the same time, breathing deeply before sleeping, eating without excess, measuring his heart rate and recording his sleep.

At first it was a challenge; then, a source of pride. Today he works as an emotional coach in a rehabilitation center. It teaches other patients that physical discipline trains the mind as well. "My psychiatrist gave me lithium. I learned to give my body a liturgy".

Studies by the Harvard Mood and Exercise Project confirm that regular exercise increases BDNF, stabilizes dopamine, and strengthens circadian synchrony. Samuel showed that neuroplasticity is also conquered through movement.

50.6 Mariana, the Scientist Mother

Biologist, 39 years old, bipolar type I. Her deepest fear was pregnancy. She had read about the risk of postpartum relapse, but decided to train with an interdisciplinary team: perinatal psychiatrist, obstetrician, and family therapist. He used lamotrigine with rigorous control and maintained sleep hygiene.

Months after giving birth, she wrote a blog about motherhood and mental health that inspired thousands of women. "I'm not a bipolar mother. I'm a mother aware of my biology". Her story changed the public conversation about pregnancy and bipolar.

Medical evidence confirms that, with planning and monitoring, motherhood and stability are compatible. Mariana showed that scientific knowledge can also be an act of love.

50.7 Daniel, the Philosopher of Inner Balance

Philosophy professor, 55 years old. He experienced mixed episodes and alcohol abuse. Recovery came when he understood that his mind needed silence. He began to meditate, not as a spiritual escape, but as brain training.

Mindfulness practice reduced their anxiety and impulsivity. He taught again, this time on philosophy and the neuroscience of consciousness. "I don't look for God outside anymore. I look for it in the act of breathing without fear".

The functional resonances of meditators like Daniel show less amygdalar activation and greater prefrontal connectivity: the brain trained in conscious attention learns to live without inner storm.

50.8 Conclusions

A clear pattern emerges in these stories: recovery does not depend on the type of drug, but on the alliance between science, discipline and purpose. All successful patients share six fundamental axes:

- rational adherence,
- stable circadian rhythm,
- permanent psychoeducation,
- emotional support network,
- clear life purpose,
- serene acceptance of vulnerability.

True strength does not consist in eliminating the disease, but in living with it from a state of lucidity.

Neuroscience confirms it: the stable brain changes its connectivity as much as the diseased brain. During prolonged recovery, the ventromedial prefrontal cortex and anterior insula —areas of self-awareness and empathy— strengthen your communication.

Stability leaves a structural imprint:

- thought becomes slower,
- emotion more predictable,
- identity more coherent.

Recovery doesn't just reorganize neurons: it reorganizes the meaning of existence.

The psychiatrist, in this process, is not an external observer, but a witness to the rebirth. Every stable session, every well-achieved adjustment, every smile after a relapse is a victory shared between biology and will. In this silent interaction between the molecule and the word, the miracle of modern psychiatry is woven: the return of the person to his or her own axis.

The stories of recovery are, at heart, contemporary parables about the human capacity to rebuild itself. They remind us:

- that even a vulnerable brain can become wise,
- that chemistry can coexist with the soul, and that stability —far from being boring— is an advanced form of art.

In bipolar disorder, every stormless day is an invisible masterpiece. Every night of restful sleep, an act of biological resistance. Every patient who learns to listen to their mind without fear is, in fact, writing a new chapter in the history of human emotional evolution.

Hope, when it becomes a habit, ceases to be a desire: it becomes a method. And in the realm of bipolarity, each serene dawn is not just another day, but an intimate victory over chaos, a living testimony that the light —even if it takes time— always returns (Figure 49).

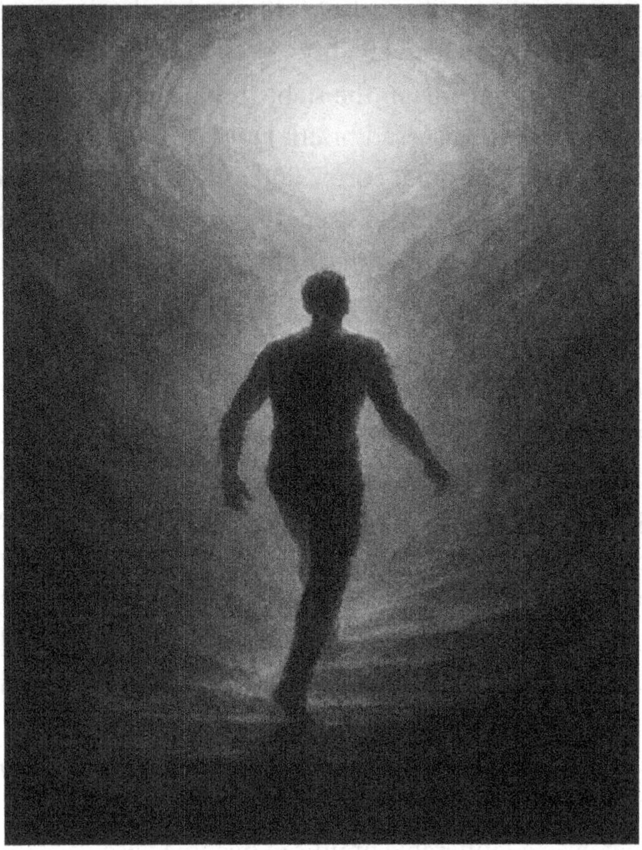

Figure 49. The figure ascending into the light represents the rebirth of stability from the darkness: the instant when science and spirit come together in recovery.

PART X.
Treatment According Population Group

CHAPTER 51
Bipolar in Women: Hormonal Cycle, Pregnancy and Postpartum

Hormones do not cause bipolarity, but they modulate its expression.

51.1 Introduction

The female body is a neuroendocrine symphony, and in bipolar disorder that music can become more sensitive, more intense, more vulnerable to changes in the environment. A woman's hormonal biology directly influences affective regulation, the clinical expression of the disorder and the response to treatments. Understanding this cyclical language does not mean pathologizing it, but integrating it into the neurochemical map of the mind.

Women with bipolar disorder do not live a single biology, but several overlapping ones: that of their reproductive hormones, that of their neurotransmitters and that of their emotional history. Each of these layers modulates mood, sleep, and self-perception. For this reason, treatment in women requires precision that goes beyond diagnostic manuals: it requires clinical art, endocrine empathy and personalized listening.

51.2 Menstrual Cycle

During the menstrual cycle, estrogen and progesterone levels change dramatically. Estrogen increases the availability of serotonin and dopamine, which boosts energy, focus, and well-being. Progesterone, on the other hand, increases GABAergic activity, promoting calmness, but also drowsiness and melancholy.

In bipolar women, these oscillations can amplify affective variations and, in sensitive cases, precipitate episodes. The phenomenon is known as bipolar premenstrual dysphoric disorder, a subtype where the days leading up to menstruation act as neurochemical catalysts for mood swings.

51.3 Pregnancy

During pregnancy, balance is redefined. The maternal brain enters a phase of intense neuroplasticity: circuits of empathy, attention and emotional memory are reorganized. However, in women with bipolar vulnerability, abrupt discontinuation of medication, insomnia, and perinatal stress can trigger episodes.

The risk of relapse during pregnancy and postpartum rises by up to 40% if not properly planned. The key is prevention rather than failure, maintaining a risk-benefit approach, and working with an interdisciplinary team.

In the reproductive stage, the main challenge is adherence. Many women stop treatment for fear of harming the baby, not understanding that emotional relapse without treatment can be more dangerous than supervised medication.

Preconception education is vital: informing, planning, adjusting doses and creating an emergency plan for emotional changes during pregnancy or postpartum. Women should feel part of their treatment, not victims of it.

Mood stabilizers such as lamotrigine and lithium may be used under close monitoring. Lamotrigine is considered one of the safest options during pregnancy, especially in women with a predominance of depression.

Lithium requires close follow-up, with serum levels measured every three weeks and adjustment before delivery to avoid neonatal toxicity. Atypical antipsychotics, such as quetiapine, are reserved for acute phases with clear clinical criteria. The guiding principle is not to "suspend everything", but to "personalize everything".

51.4 Postpartum

The postpartum period represents one of the most risky moments in the entire female bipolar path. The abrupt drop in estrogen and progesterone levels after childbirth generates a neurochemical storm that affects even women without a previous diagnosis. In those who already have a history of bipolar, this dysregulation can precipitate a manic, depressive, or mixed episode, often in the first two weeks. The phenomenon is known as bipolar postpartum psychosis, a psychiatric emergency that requires immediate hospitalization and stabilizing treatment with antipsychotics or lithium under medical supervision.

Beyond biology, the postpartum period implies a profound symbolic change: identity is reconfigured, time is fragmented, sleep is interrupted, and the body —which was a container of life— now feels exhausted. In this area, mental vulnerability can flourish without guilt, but so can resilience. Family and therapeutic accompaniment is essential: the mother needs to be cared for in order to be able to care (Figure 50).

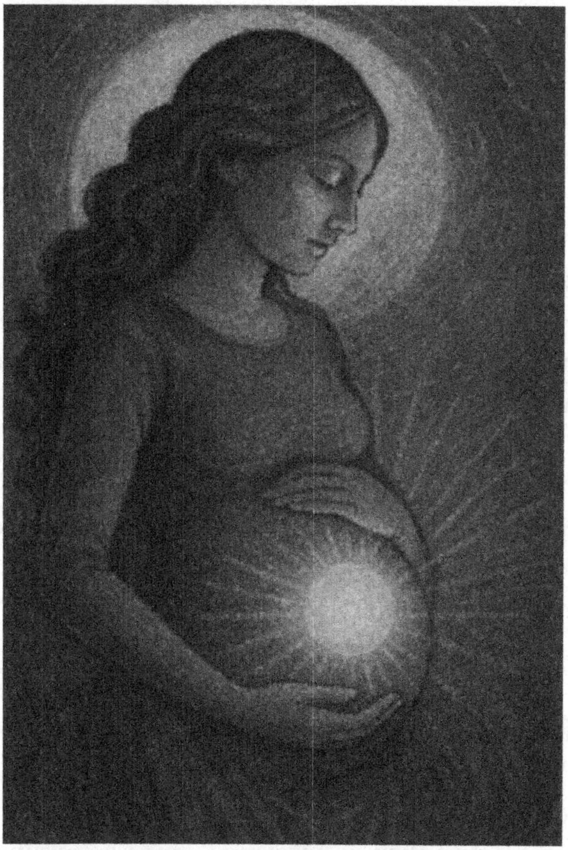

Figure 50. The golden light inside the mother represents hormonal harmony, neuro-emotional balance, and the deep wisdom of the female body.

51.5 Menopause

In menopause, the panorama is transformed again. The progressive decrease in estrogen and sleep disturbance can reactivate depressive or mixed symptoms. However, many women also experience an emotional maturity that allows for better self-regulation.

Evidence suggests that hormone replacement therapy may be helpful in some cases, but should be assessed on an individual basis, especially if there is a history of thrombosis, cancer, or cardiovascular risk. At this stage, psychotherapeutic therapies, meditation, physical exercise and sleep regulation become fundamental pillars.

51.6 Conclusions

The emotional dimension of the female hormonal cycle goes beyond the laboratory. Every transition—menarche, pregnancy, postpartum, menopause—involves a redesign of the self.

In women with bipolarity, these stages are not weaknesses, but moments of profound readjustment, where identity is renewed and consciousness expands. Understanding your own rhythm is a form of biological autonomy.

Science confirms it: estrogens modulate the sensitivity of dopaminergic receptors in the striatum and progesterone acts on GABA-A receptors, which generates calmness or sedation. Serotonin and cortisol also fluctuate, affecting sleep, appetite, and anxiety. This framework turns women into a living laboratory of hormonal adaptation, where balance is conquered with self-knowledge.

From a humanistic perspective, every woman who manages to go through pregnancy, postpartum or menopause without losing her axis is a master of internal synchrony. There is no treatment more powerful than understanding your own body, and no medication more effective than an informed, empathetic support network. Contemporary psychiatry must learn to look at the female brain not as a territory of risk, but as a biological orchestra of resilience.

Bipolarity in women is a metaphor for nature itself: cyclical, changing, intense, but profoundly capable of self-regulation when offered knowledge, rest, and respect. In it dwells the purest evidence that life, even in the midst of disorder, always tends towards harmony.

CHAPTER 52
Childhood and Adolescent Bipolarity: Early Diagnoses and Controversies

To diagnose in time is to protect development;
not labeling childhood.

52.1 Introduction

To speak of bipolar disorder in childhood and adolescence is to enter one of the most complex and debated territories of contemporary psychiatry. For decades, bipolar disorder was believed to be an adult-only illness. However, the latest research shows that the neurobiology of affective control can begin in childhood.

What was previously interpreted as "difficult behavior" or "stages of rebellion" may, in some cases, be the early expression of a mind that has not yet learned to regulate its neurochemical oscillations.

The clinical challenge lies in differentiating the normal changes in emotional development —typical of childhood and adolescence— from the persistent pathological symptoms that indicate bipolar vulnerability.

All children change their moods; but the bipolar child does not fluctuate on a whim, but because of brain dysregulation. Their episodes don't last minutes: they last days, sometimes weeks. Their energy isn't just enthusiasm: it's dopaminergic overload. Their sadness isn't just frustration: it's a profound decline in motivation and social connection.

52.2 Childhood

Neuroimaging studies reveal that in children with bipolar predisposition there is a tonsillar hyperreactivity in the face of emotional stimuli and a delayed maturation of the prefrontal cortex, the region responsible for modulating impulses. This dissonance between emotion and control generates a brain in "desynchronized mode": it feels before thinking, it acts before evaluating. Therefore, the diagnosis should not be based only on behavior, but on a comprehensive reading of the child's neurocognitive, family and evolutionary profile.

In clinical practice, symptoms usually manifest differently than in adults. Instead of classic episodes of euphoria or depression, children may exhibit chronic irritability, emotional outbursts, intermittent aggression, rapid mood swings, sleep disturbances, and low tolerance for frustration.

This pattern has been described as disruptive mood dysregulation disorder (DMDD), a category introduced in the DSM-5 to avoid overdiagnosis of bipolar disorder in the pediatric population. However, some experts argue that in a subset of these children, DMDD is simply the prelude to bipolar disorder in adolescence or adulthood.

Genetics provides more clarity than controversy. Studies of twins and families show that if one parent has bipolar disorder, the risk in the children increases 10 to 20 times. It is not the disease that is inherited, but the sensitivity of the limbic system to dopaminergic and circadian changes.

This predisposition is activated by environmental factors: stress, irregular sleep, family conflicts or childhood trauma. The combination of biological vulnerability and chaotic environments can trigger the first affective episode before the age of 15.

Early diagnosis is a double-edged sword. Done wisely, it can save a life; done lightly, it can stigmatize a childhood. For this reason, psychiatrists specialising in the child population must act rigorously, avoiding premature labels and opting for longitudinal observation.

Family history, sleep pattern, stress response, and academic performance are just as important as visible emotion. In many cases, the first clue appears at school: teachers who notice emotional hyperactivity, persistent irritability, or periods of alternating isolation and awesomeness.

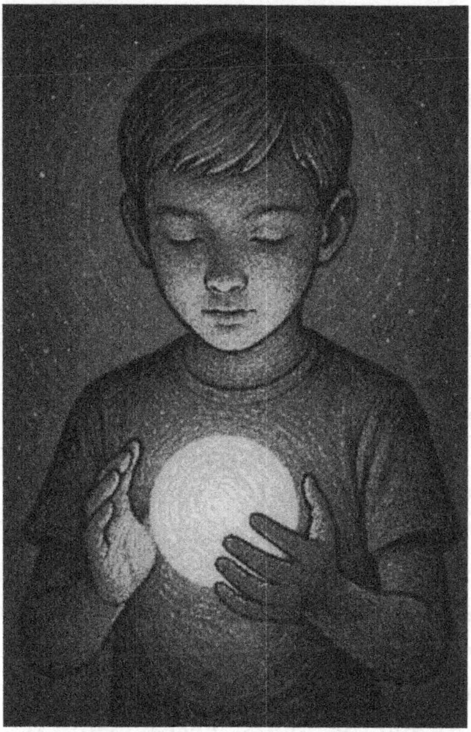

Figure 51. The child holding the light represents emotional self-regulation, neural growth, and the awakening of consciousness in early bipolarity.

52.3 Adolescence

In adolescence, the picture becomes more recognizable. The bipolar young person alternates periods of enthusiasm, creativity, sociability and high energy with stages of apathy, insomnia, disinterest and thoughts of uselessness.

The risks multiply: substance use, sexual impulsivity, lack of sleep and constant digital exposure act as triggers for dopaminergic circuits. The adolescent brain is already hyperplastic and sensitive to reward; adding an affective disorder makes it a perfect storm.

Treatment must be adapted to this sensitivity. Mood stabilizers, such as lamotrigine or lithium, are used with lower doses and close monitoring. Atypical antipsychotics —quetiapine, aripiprazole, lurasidone— may be useful for acute control, always under medical supervision. But no drug replaces emotional education: the child or adolescent must learn to recognize their early signs, regulate their sleep, structure their routine and verbalize their emotions. Cognitive-behavioral psychotherapy and family therapy are equivalent pillars to pharmacological treatment.

52.4 Psychoeducation for Parents

One of the greatest advances in child psychiatry has been psychoeducation for parents. When the family understands that mood swings are not a lack of discipline, but biological symptoms, the emotional climate of the home changes radically. Punishment is replaced by accompaniment, criticism by empathic observation, guilt by cooperation. The family becomes the child's first stabilizer.

Longitudinal studies show that children treated early and with good adherence have a more favorable outcome: fewer hospitalizations, lower risk of suicide, and better school performance. The key is to accompany development without suffocating it, to balance structure and freedom, science and affection.

Controversies persist. Some sectors of psychiatry criticize early diagnosis for fear of overmedicating or labeling. Others argue that ignoring symptoms for fear of diagnosis is also a form of negligence. The truth, as almost always, is in the middle ground: evaluate with prudence, intervene with humanity, accompany with continuity.

52.5 Conclusions

In childhood and adolescent bipolarity, it is not only about stabilizing a brain: it is about protecting a story. Each child with affective dysregulation is a potential adult who can shine if he is taught to manage his energy without losing his essence. Early prevention not only prevents future crises, but also preserves the possibility of a creative and fulfilling destiny.

The future of paediatric psychiatry will be inclusive. The new tools – genetic biomarkers, sleep analysis, artificial intelligence applied to behavioural monitoring – will make it possible to distinguish more precisely between evolutionary and pathological instability.

But no technology will replace the human gaze capable of reading the soul behind the symptom. That gaze, when compassionate and scientific at the same time, can change the course of an entire life.

Childhood bipolarity is not the end of innocence; it is the opportunity to learn to take care of the mind from the earliest years. And every adolescent who manages to find balance between their energy, their thinking, and their identity is living proof that neuroplasticity can also be called hope.

CHAPTER 53
Bipolar Disorder in Older Age: Medical Complications and Cognition

In old age, bipolarity does not scream: it whispers.

53.1 Bipolarity that Ages: A Language Different from the Mood

In old age, bipolarity manifests itself in a different language. The emotional storms of the past can be transformed into persistent drizzles or, sometimes, into silences that confuse diagnosis with wear and tear. Aging modifies neurochemistry, synaptic plasticity, and the way the brain regulates emotional energy. The psychiatrist must learn to read in the wrinkle what was previously read in the impulse: the mood no longer explodes, it is extinguished; he does not always scream, sometimes he fades away.

53.2 Geriatric Bipolarity

Geriatric bipolarity is not a simple extension of juvenile bipolarity: it is a neurodegenerative, vascular and cognitive phenomenon. Studies show that about 10% of bipolar patients over 60 years of age have mild cognitive impairment or dementia associated with their affective history.

Repeated episodes, prolonged exposure to oxidative stress, and silent micro-infarctions can disrupt frontolimbic circuits, reducing cognitive flexibility and working memory. The result is a mind that retains emotion, but loses precision in response. Brain aging with bipolarity involves three dimensions: neurobiological, medical, and existential.

53.3 Neurobiological Dimension: When Mood Slows Down

In the neurobiological dimension, dopamine and serotonin decrease, cortical metabolism slows down, and neurogenesis mechanisms are reduced. This explains why many older patients experience less intense mania, but more prolonged depressive episodes, with apathy, psychomotor slowness and anhedonia. Neural plasticity no longer responds with the same speed, but retains the ability to adapt if adequately stimulated with therapy, exercise and vital sense.

53.4 Medical Dimension: Comorbidities and Pharmacological Fragility

In the medical dimension, comorbidities become protagonists. Hypertension, diabetes, kidney failure, hypothyroidism, and cardiovascular disease modify the pharmacokinetics of mood stabilizers.

Lithium, considered a gold drug, requires closer monitoring: kidney and thyroid function should be assessed every three months, and doses adjusted for changes in creatinine clearance.

Antipsychotics should be used with caution, as they increase the risk of falls, sedation, and metabolic syndrome. In many cases, lamotrigine and lurasidone are safer options due to their lower metabolic impact and better cognitive profile.

53.5 Cognitive Dimension: Affective Deterioration Without Loss of Humanity

The cognitive dimension is the most subtle and the most painful. Many patients report "loss of mental agility", "clouding" or difficulty in organizing ideas. It is not always dementia, but the combination of natural aging, vascular micro-lesions and the cumulative effects of affective episodes.

Research in geriatric neuropsychiatry has identified a specific syndrome: "affective cognitive impairment", characterized by decreased episodic memory and sustained attention, but with preservation of social judgment and empathy. It is the mind that forgets details, but retains humanity.

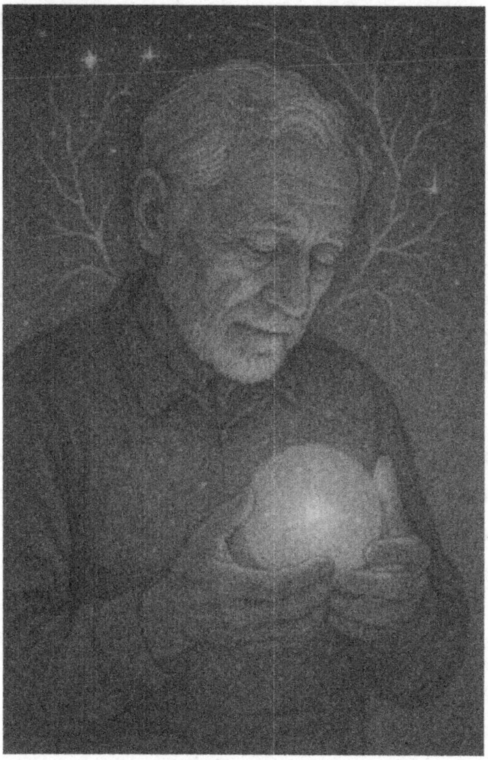

Figure 52. The old man holding the light represents serenity, wisdom, and the peaceful balance between mind and time..

53.6 Therapeutic Principles in the Elderly

The treatment of bipolar in the elderly should be slower, gentler and continuous. Sudden changes in medication or rapid reductions can cause serious decompensation. It is recommended to prioritize drugs with low interaction potential, maintain stable plasma levels, and perform periodic polypharmacy check-ups. Coordination with internal medicine, neurology, and geriatrics is not optional, but essential.

53.7 The Environment and Attachments as Neurobiological Stabilizers

Trying is not enough: you have to accompany. Loneliness is the most powerful negative stabilizer in old age. The brain needs bonds as much as it needs medication. Cognitive stimulation, social participation, music therapy, adapted physical activity and existential psychotherapy reduce relapses and improve affective memory. The aged mind, when it feels useful, produces dopamine again.

53.8 Cumulative Grief and Meaning Therapy

In the psychological field, bipolar geriatric depression has a particular nuance: accumulated grief. The patient does not cry only for the present, but for everything lost: people, time, body, projects.

Therapy must integrate the past as a legacy, not as a weight. Turning biography into wisdom is a form of treatment. Logotherapy and reminiscence therapy are especially valuable at this stage: they help to rebuild meaning and dignity in the midst of aging.

53.9 Spirituality and Lucid Serenity in Old Age

Spirituality —understood not as religion, but as a transcendent connection— takes on special relevance. Many patients find stability in rediscovering a purpose that transcends the personal: love for grandchildren, teaching, art, faith, or simply serene contemplation of life. Hope in old age is not euphoria: it is lucid serenity.

53.10 Late Neuroplasticity and Peace Learning

Neuroscience backs it up. Studies with functional resonance show that meditation and gratitude increase connectivity between the dorsolateral prefrontal cortex and the precuneus, regions related to introspection and acceptance. In other words, the elderly brain can continue to learn peace.

53.11 Emotional Wisdom and Mature Resilience

Bipolarity in old age also invites us to reflect on the history of the mind. Each episode overcome leaves traces: some scars, but also learnings. Many older patients report that although the intensity of moods decreases, their emotional wisdom increases. "I don't fear my dark days anymore", they say, "because I know they pass". That awareness, won over decades of struggle, is treatment's highest achievement: a form of mature resilience.

53.12 The Clinic as a Testimony of Life

In clinical practice, every consultation with a bipolar elderly patient is a lesson in time, patience, and humility. The doctor ceases to be a regulator of medicines to become a witness to a biography.

The objective is no longer only to stabilize the mood, but to preserve identity, memory and meaning. Because in old age, healing is not always about eliminating symptoms: sometimes it is teaching how to live in balance with them.

53.13 Old Age As a Chapter of Psychiatric Wisdom

The elderly and bipolarity are not inevitable enemies. They are two realities that, when embraced with understanding and science, can give rise to a form of serene wisdom: a mind that has known euphoria and sadness, but chooses calm as a form of wisdom. In this balance between neurochemistry and philosophy, between memory and biology, old age becomes the most human chapter of psychiatry.

CHAPTER 54
Bipolar Disorder with ADHD, Anxiety, Trauma, or Autism Spectrum

The mind is not organized by isolated diagnoses,
but by overlapping networks.

54.1 Introduction

The human mind rarely obeys the limits of a diagnosis. In clinical practice, bipolar disorder does not usually present alone: it shares space, territory, and neurocircuitry with other disorders such as ADHD, anxiety disorders, complex psychological trauma, and autism spectrum conditions.

Understanding these intersections not only broadens the psychiatrist's view, but redefines the way we understand the contemporary mind: a web of memories, impulses, and defenses that interact in the same brain.

54.2 Bipolarity and ADHD: Energy without Focus

Attention deficit hyperactivity disorder (ADHD) is one of the most common comorbidities in bipolar patients, especially in those whose first episode appears before the age of 20. Both conditions share dysfunctions in the dopaminergic and noradrenergic systems, with an alteration of the frontostriatal circuit. In clinical terms, symptoms of impulsivity, distractibility, restlessness, and low tolerance for frustration overlap.

The diagnostic challenge lies in differentiating the chronic hyperactivity of ADHD from the episodic energy of mania. In ADHD, the pattern is continuous and appears from childhood; in bipolarity, it is intermittent and alternates with phases of dejection. Treatment requires balance: psychostimulants can worsen mania if the mood is not stabilized first.

Therefore, the golden rule is to treat bipolar first and then attentional, with strategies that integrate mood stabilizers, psychoeducation, and behavioral therapy focused on organization, planning, and emotional regulation.

54.3 Bipolarity and Anxiety: the Alarm System on Fire

The coexistence of generalized anxiety, panic, or obsessive-compulsive disorder with bipolar creates a state of chronic hyperalertness. The limbic system, particularly the amygdala, remains overexcited, which enhances depressive relapses and prolonged insomnia.

The anxious bipolar patient fears both euphoria and fall, lives anticipating the lack of control, and that anticipation becomes a second disorder. Treatment should address the GABAergic and serotonergic axis without activating mania. Short-term anxiolytics, cognitive-behavioral therapies focused on tolerance to uncertainty, and neurophysiological mindfulness have shown efficacy.

Controlled breathing, gradual exposure, and autonomic nervous system retraining techniques help turn off the "brain alarm" that keeps the patient in a state of war with themselves.

54.4 Bipolarity and Trauma: the Memory that Does not Sleep

Psychological trauma alters the same circuits as bipolarity: amygdala, hippocampus, and medial prefrontal cortex. When a traumatized brain develops bipolar disorder, emotional memories are reactivated with each mood swing. Euphoria can bring flashbacks disguised as power; depression, guilt and paralysis.

The modern concept of post-traumatic bipolar disorder recognizes that early events of abuse, neglect, or violence increase dopaminergic sensitivity and disrupt circadian rhythms. Treatment should integrate pharmacotherapy with trauma processing therapy, such as EMDR (eye movement desensitization and reprocessing) or sociomotor therapies, as well as somatic work to reconnect body and mind.

The key is for the patient to understand that their reactivity is not moral weakness, but physiological memory. Every crisis is an attempt by the body to process what the soul could not verbalize.

54.5 Bipolarity and the Autism Spectrum: Two Different Ways of Feeling the World

In some patients, especially young men and women with mild or undiagnosed autism, bipolar presents with atypical features: extreme emotions, rigidity in routines, and difficulties in social interpretation.

The autism spectrum shares with bipolar disorder alterations in the connectivity between the medial prefrontal cortex and the temporal regions, which affects affective regulation and the reading of the emotional environment.

In practice, these patients can be mistaken for "cold" or "unempathetic" bipolars, when in fact their emotion is regulated by a different sensory system.

Treatment should focus on the patient's sensory understanding: avoid overstimulation and prioritize structured therapies and family psychoeducation. Soft stabilizers and environmental routine are essential to avoid imbalances.

54.6 The Polyphonic Mind

In all these pictures, the bipolar mind becomes a polyphonic system where different disorders dialogue and influence each other. It is not a question of silencing a voice, but of harmonizing them. Each comorbidity requires a different therapeutic order, but they all share the same goal: to integrate, not fragment.

The contemporary psychiatrist must act as a neurochemical conductor, adjusting the volume of each system without shutting down the overall melody. That melody, deep down, is the patient's story: their defenses, their learnings, their grief, their attempts to find meaning within the chaos.

Neuroscience confirms that brains with multiple diagnoses show greater interconnectivity between networks —the default mode, the executive control network, and the salience network—which gives them intense emotional sensitivity and, paradoxically, superior creative capacity when they are stable. The same mind that suffers most deeply is also the one that can create, understand, and love most deeply.

54.7 Conclusions

The treatment of bipolar disorder with comorbidities is not only pharmacological: it is a complex architecture where biology, history and context are intertwined. In the patient with ADHD, anxiety, trauma or autism, the goal is not to erase labels, but to build a functional balance where each diagnosis finds its place within a mind that remains one.

Because, in the end, beyond names and manuals, every bipolar human being with multiple diagnoses seeks the same thing: a point of inner stillness where chemistry and consciousness are reconciled (Figure 53).

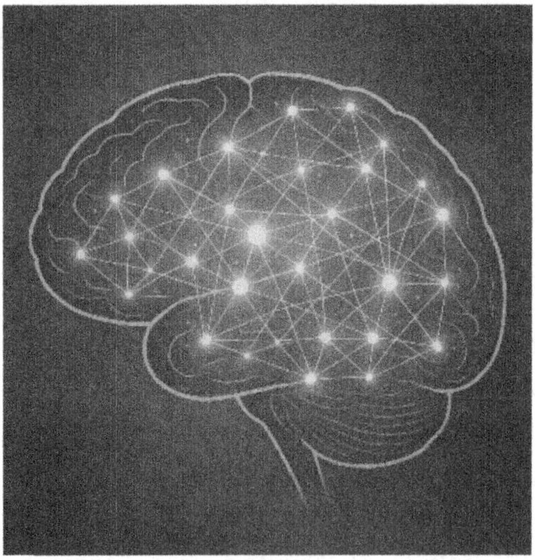

Figure 53. The interconnected lights symbolize the harmony of complex neural systems, where bipolarity, ADHD, anxiety, trauma, and autism converge in an integrated mind.

PART XI.
Where to Go for Help?

CHAPTER 55
Mexico: Psychiatric Hospitals, NGO, Digital Platforms and Crisis Lines

Asking for help is not giving up:
it is activating the network that sustains life.

55.1 Seeking Help as an Act of Clinical and Human Wisdom

Seeking help should not be an act of desperation, but of wisdom. In Mexico, thousands of people with bipolar disorder face the challenge of finding timely, comprehensive, and accessible care.

The country has made progress in creating public and community mental health networks, but the gap between need and care remains wide. However, behind this difficulty there is also a silent network of professionals, institutions and civil organizations that day by day accompany, contain and guide those who are going through a crisis.

55.2 National Mental Health System: Public Care Structure

The first level of care is represented by the National Mental Health System (SISAME), which includes psychiatric hospitals, outpatient units and Comprehensive Mental Health Centers (CISAME). These centers, distributed in several regions of the country, offer psychiatric evaluation, psychotherapy, pharmacological management and family psychoeducation free of charge or at low cost.

55.3 Psychiatric Hospitals and National Referral Institutions

Among the most recognized institutions are the following:

- **"Fray Bernardino Álvarez" Psychiatric Hospital (Mexico City):** the oldest in the country, with hospitalization, emergency and outpatient services. National reference for affective and psychotic disorders.

- **"Juan N. Navarro" Children's Psychiatric Hospital:** specialized in the care of children and adolescents with mood, behavior and neurodevelopmental disorders.
- **National Institute of Psychiatry "Ramón de la Fuente Muñiz":** center for research and advanced clinical care; offers programs on bipolar disorder, depression, addictions and psychoeducation.
- **Psychiatric Hospital of Yucatán and Civil Hospital of Guadalajara:** pioneers in community care and training of specialists in psychiatry.
- **Youth Integration Centers (CIJ):** although focused on addictions, they provide free psychological care to young people with depressive, anxious or bipolar symptoms.

55.4 CISAME and Decentralized Community Care

At the community level, Comprehensive Mental Health Centers (CISAME) play a crucial role. Multidisciplinary teams of psychiatrists, psychologists, nurses and social workers work in them. They are found in states such as Veracruz, Puebla, Oaxaca, Chihuahua, Sonora and Nuevo León. They offer continuous care, family counseling and social reintegration programs.

55.5 Digital Platforms and Telepsychiatry in Mexico

Access to mental health in Mexico has also been digitized. Several online platforms have emerged to connect patients with certified professionals:

- Telethon Mental Health, with free psychological care via video call.
- Telegalenos.com, a telepsychiatry and emotional health project that offers consultations in Spanish and English with specialists from different regions.
- Psicólogos.org.mx, Doctoralia, and MindCare Mexico, platforms with filters by specialty, location, and cost.

- The National Institute of Psychiatry's National Telepsychiatry Network, which connects rural hospitals with psychiatrists in real time.

55.6 Crisis Lines and Immediate Attention

In emergency situations, it is essential to know the crisis and immediate attention lines, available 24 hours a day:

- SAPTEL (Distance Psychological Support Service): 800 472 7835. Free, confidential and available all year round.
- Lifeline (CONADIC): 800 911 2000. Psychological and psychiatric support for substance use, depression and emotional crises.
- National Emergencies: 911, with referral to mental health and psychological first aid units.
- Locatel CDMX: 55 5658 1111. It offers medical and psychological guidance.
- UNAM Community Psychology: 800 999 6266. Free care by supervised professionals.

55.7 NGO and Civil Associations: Support Beyond the System

In parallel, various NGO and civil associations work tirelessly to make mental health visible and accompany patients and their families:

- Mexican Foundation for Mental Health (FMSM): promotes public education and the fight against stigma.
- Fundación Bipolar México: organization dedicated to information, support groups and educational campaigns.
- Asociación Voz Pro Salud Mental (VPSM): offers workshops and counseling for relatives of patients with affective disorders.
- Red Pro Cuidados Comunitarios: promotes the creation of safe spaces for patients with chronic psychiatric conditions.

These associations offer education, support groups, family workshops and anti-stigma campaigns.

55.8 Family, Community and Culture as Protective Factors

The Mexican social fabric, with its strong sense of community, represents an invaluable opportunity: the family and the community are the first pillars of prevention. Family psychoeducation, support groups and participation in specialized social networks help to transform the patient's loneliness into collective accompaniment.

Mexican culture, so rich in bonds, can become a therapeutic ally. Spaces for faith, art, music, and volunteerism offer meaning, structure, and connection. Every person who listens, every family who gets informed, every community that breaks the silence is contributing to the mental health of the country.

55.9 Towards a More Humane and Accessible Mental Health

Access to help is not always immediate, but it is becoming more and more possible. Mexico is moving towards a more humane, digital and decentralized model, where asking for help is no longer an act of shame, but of courage. In a country where so many stories coexist with resilience, mental health is beginning to occupy the place it always deserved: the center of life (Figure 54).

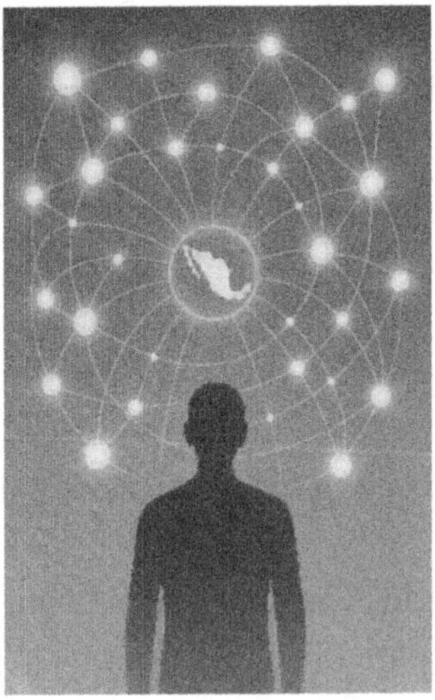

Figure 54. The luminous network symbolizes the expansion of hospitals, crisis lines, and community programs that come together for mental health in Mexico.

CHAPTER 56
Spain: Public Services, Support Associations and Community Centers

Mental health is built in community.

56.1 Spain and the Community Model of Mental Health

Spain has built one of the most solid and humanized public mental health systems in Europe. Unlike purely hospital models, the Spanish approach privileges community care, family integration and multidisciplinary coordination.

For people living with bipolar disorder, this translates into closer, more continuous and personalized access, where stability is conceived not only as chemical balance, but as social and relational well-being.

56.2 National Health System: Public Access and Continuity of Care

The Spanish health system, through the National Health System (SNS), guarantees free access to psychiatric and psychological care within the public network. Patients can go to their family doctor, who refers them to the Mental Health Centers (CSM) depending on the health area.

These centres are staffed by teams made up of psychiatrists, clinical psychologists, specialist nurses and occupational therapists. Care is free, and in many cases includes home visits, individual or group psychotherapy, and reintegration programs.

56.3 Hospitals and Referral Centres for Bipolar Disorder

Among the centers and hospitals of national reference are:

- Hospital Clínic de Barcelona: with its Bipolar Disorders Unit, a leader in research and personalised treatment.

- Gregorio Marañón University Hospital (Madrid): pioneer in comprehensive care and family psychoeducation programs.
- Hospital de la Santa Creu i Sant Pau (Barcelona): recognized for its interdisciplinary approach and its participation in European projects on affective neuroscience.
- Virgen del Rocío Hospital (Seville) and University Hospital of Valencia: with community mental health and relapse prevention programs.
- Carlos III Health Institute: main research entity in neuroscience and mental public health.

56.4 Day Centres: the Bridge between Hospital and Everyday Life

The Spanish model incorporates an essential figure: the Day Centre, where patients with bipolar disorder or major depression can go during the day to participate in workshops, psychotherapy, cognitive training and artistic or work activities. These centers function as bridges between hospitalization and daily life, which reduces relapses and strengthens the autonomy of patients.

56.5 Patient and Family Associations: Accompaniment and Psychoeducation

Patient and family associations play a key role in education and emotional support. Some of the most important are:

- Bipolar Association of Madrid (ABM): offers support groups, family counseling and campaigns against stigma.
- Catalan Association of Bipolar Disorder (ACTB): a benchmark in psychoeducation and self-help programmes throughout Catalonia.
- Bipolar Association of Eastern Andalusia: promotes training and suicide prevention activities.
- FEAFES (Spanish Confederation of Mental Health): national network of associations with a presence in all autonomous communities.

- Bipolar World Foundation: organizes conferences, outreach programs and peer support.

56.6 The Family as an Active Therapeutic Agent

Family psychoeducation, which is highly developed in Spain, is considered part of the standard treatment. Family members learn to identify signs of relapse, to manage communication and to accompany without overprotecting. The family is not seen as a source of conflict, but as an active therapeutic agent.

56.7 Digital Platforms and Emotional Support Lines

Spain has also made progress in the digitalisation of mental health, with multiple accessible platforms:

- Mental Health Spain (www.consaludmental.org): information portal and national directory of resources.
- Psychology at Home and PsicoGlobal: certified virtual consultations.
- "Prevensuic" App and "SAM" App of the Ministry of Health, designed to detect crisis risk and offer immediate assistance.
- Telephone of Hope (717 003 717): free and confidential 24-hour emotional support line.
- Telephone 024: national suicide prevention line.

These tools expand access and allow for early intervention.

56.8 Crisis Care: Mobile Teams and Rapid Response

In terms of crisis intervention, Spain has become an example of rapid and interdisciplinary response. In most cities there are mobile mental health teams, which go to homes or public spaces when a patient goes into decompensation. This strategy avoids unnecessary hospitalizations and promotes containment in the patient's natural environment.

56.9 The Three Pillars of the Spanish Community Model

The Spanish Community model is based on three pillars:

1. Accessibility: no patient is left without care due to lack of resources (Figure 55).
2. Continuity: the teams accompany you throughout the process, even in phases of stability.
3. Destigmatization: Mental illness is treated as just another medical condition, not as a social label.

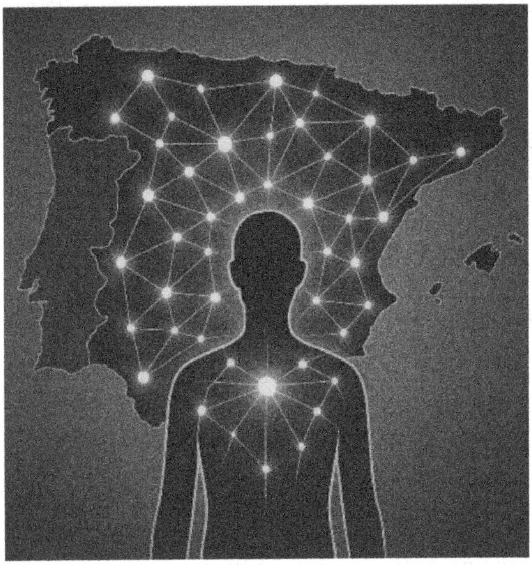

Figure 55. The connected lights throughout Spain represent the harmony between public care, community networks and individual healing.

56.10 Precision Research and Psychiatry

In addition, Spanish neuropsychiatric research is among the most advanced in the world. The projects of the Hospital Clínic and the Carlos III Institute have identified biological markers of bipolar disorder, such as alterations in the connectivity of the frontolimbic network, circadian rhythms and plasma levels of brain-derived neurotrophic factor (BDNF). This precision science is enabling a more personalized, less pharmacocentric, and more humane approach.

56.11 Culture, Community and Dignity of Care

Culturally, Spain combines science and compassion. The health system, together with social and family networks, generates an ecosystem where the bipolar patient can recover not only stability, but also the dignity of living with others. The autonomous communities are increasingly promoting spaces for dialogue, art, and coexistence, understanding that mental health flourishes in integration, not in isolation.

56.12 Mental Health as Shared Well-being

Ultimately, seeking help in Spain means entering a system that believes in the possibility of full recovery, where emotional balance is achieved with the same seriousness with which a physical illness is treated. In a country where empathy is expressed in everyday language, mental health is experienced for what it truly is: a form of shared well-being.

CHAPTER 57
United States: Community Clinics, Bilingual Resources & Emergency Services

In a fragmented system,
Knowing where to seek help can save a life.

57.1 Introduction

The United States is a country of great contrasts, not only in its geography and culture, but also in access to mental health. For those living with bipolar disorder, the U.S. system may be both one of the most technologically advanced and one of the most fragmented in accessibility.

Understanding how and where to seek help is essential, especially for Spanish-speaking and immigrant communities, who face additional barriers of language, cost, and culture.

The U.S. healthcare system is decentralized: services vary by state, type of health insurance, and available local resources. Amid that diversity, however, is a strong network of community clinics, nonprofits, and crisis response systems that provide accessible care to those dealing with bipolar disorder and other emotional conditions.

57.2 Community Mental Health Clinics

The backbone of public psychiatric care in the United States is made up of Community Mental Health Centers (CMHCs). These clinics, funded by federal and state programs, offer psychiatric evaluation, psychotherapy, medication management and case coordination, often for free or at income-adjusted rates.

Some of the most important community programs are:

- SAMHSA (Substance Abuse and Mental Health Services Administration): Offers a national directory of public and nonprofit clinics in findtreatment.gov.
- Federally Qualified Health Centers (FQHCs): Comprehensive clinics that combine general medical care and mental health, available regardless of immigration status or health insurance.
- County Mental Health Departments: Present in every state, they provide crisis stabilization services, outpatient care, and liaison to community programs.
- National Alliance on Mental Illness (NAMI): Through its local chapters, it offers bilingual education, family support, and peer group programs for people with bipolar disorder.

In many rural or urban areas, telepsychiatry has become an indispensable bridge. Platforms such as Teladoc, Amwell, and Talkiatry make it possible to connect with psychiatrists certified in English or Spanish, expanding access to those who have transportation difficulties or live in remote regions.

57.3 Bilingual Resources and Support for Immigrants

For the Latino and immigrant population, language is one of the main barriers in seeking care. Fortunately, more and more organizations are working to close that gap:

- Mental Health America (MHA): Offers free emotional assessment tools and educational materials in Spanish.
- The Trevor Project (for LGBTQ+ youth): Provides 24-hour crisis intervention, in English and Spanish, by phone, chat, or text.
- National Latino Behavioral Health Association (NLBHA): Promotes culturally competent care and connects patients with bilingual professionals across the country.

- Telegalenos.com: Bilingual telepsychiatry network that offers consultations in English and Spanish with specialists in depression and bipolar disorder.
- American Psychological Association (APA): maintains a public database of psychologists and therapists who serve in Spanish.

There are also religious or community organizations, such as Catholic Charities, Jewish Family Services, and La Clinica del Pueblo (Washington, D.C.), which offer free or low-cost psychological counseling with a cultural focus and social sensitivity.

57.4 Crisis and Emergency Services

In situations of emotional crisis, having immediate help can save lives. The United States has a strong network of emergency mental health services:

- National Suicide Prevention and Crisis Lifeline (988): Available 24/7 in English and Spanish, connects with trained counselors across the country.
- SAMHSA National Helpline: 1-800-662-HELP (4357). Toll-free and confidential referral line for mental health and addiction treatment.
- Crisis Text Line: Text "HELLO" or "HOLA" to the 741741 for immediate bilingual emotional support.
- Mobile Crisis Teams: Available in many states, with professionals who come to the home to safely stabilize the patient.
- Hospital Emergency Rooms: By law (EMTALA), they must provide psychiatric evaluation to anyone in crisis, regardless of insurance or immigration status.

For Spanish-speaking families, knowing these numbers and sharing them in the community can make the difference between confusion and contention at a critical time.

57.5 Education, Peer Networks, and Patient Advocacy

Beyond medical treatment, long-term recovery depends on education and social support. Various organizations promote psychoeducation and empowerment:

- Depression and Bipolar Support Alliance (DBSA): Offers hundreds of free, bilingual support groups, both in-person and virtual.
- Bipolar Caregivers Alliance: helps family members improve communication, set boundaries and prevent relapse.
- Mental Health First Aid (MHFA): Trains teachers, employers, and citizens to recognize and respond to signs of emotional crisis.
- The Jed Foundation: Promotes mental health in teens and college students.
- American Foundation for Suicide Prevention (AFSP): Promotes national campaigns, survivor support, and educational programs.

57.6 Challenges and Hope

The U.S. system faces significant challenges: health insurance inequality, fragmented access, and persistence of stigma, especially in rural or minority communities. But there are signs of change.

The creation of the 988 number as a national emotional emergency line, the expansion of telemedicine and the increase in bilingual services represent a shift towards a more inclusive model. Awareness campaigns and the rise of online psychotherapy are helping to normalize help-seeking.

For immigrants and Latinos, asking for help isn't just a medical act: it's an act of bravery. It means building a bridge between cultures, breaking inherited silences and claiming the right to heal. The history of mental health in America is still being written, but its direction is clear: toward a more compassionate, more humane, and more accessible system, where emotional stability is a form of freedom. In this narrative, the search for balance becomes a profound expression of collective resilience (Figure 56).

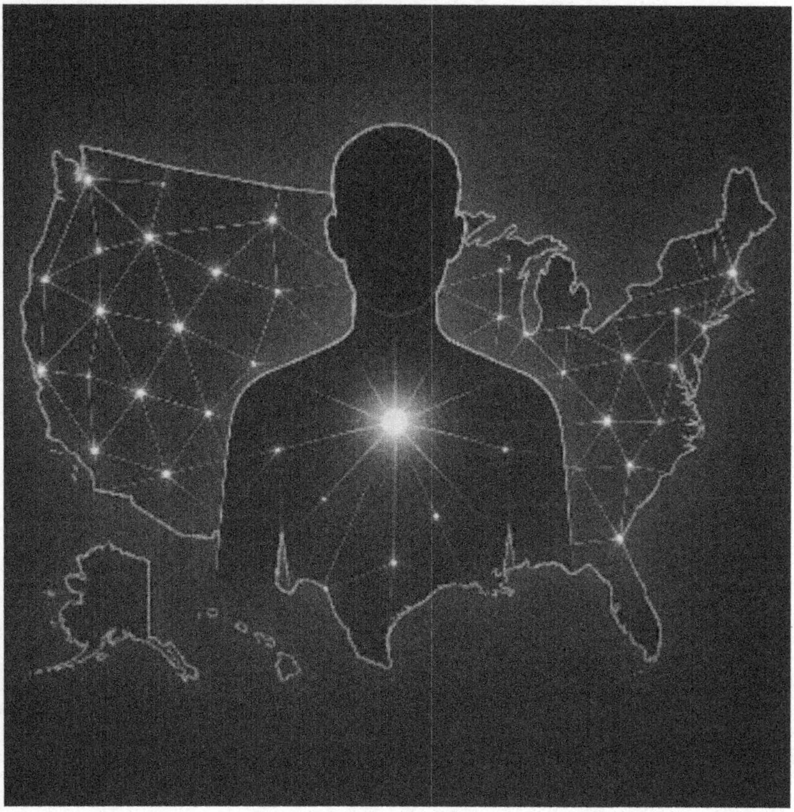

Figure 56. The central figure represents hope and the connection between mental health services across the country, united by a network of human and technological support.

PART XII.
Psychic Energy in Motion

CHAPTER 58
Table of Neurotransmitters and Associated Bipolar Symptoms

Understanding the symptoms starts with understanding the neurotransmitters.

Bipolar disorder is, first and foremost, a neurochemical orchestra. Each episode, whether of euphoria or depression, reflects a change in the dynamic balance between the brain's major neurotransmitters. To understand these substances is not to reduce the mind to chemistry, but to recognize that biology and emotional experience are two languages of the same phenomenon: psychic energy in motion.

58.1 The Bipolar Brain: Balance and Deregulation

In the brain of a person with bipolar disorder, neural communication systems work with extreme sensitivity. Changes in sleep, sunlight, stress, or hormones can modify the release or reuptake of neurotransmitters in a matter of hours, triggering intense mood swings.

Science has identified twelve major neurotransmitters involved in mood regulation and cognition. Each participates in a different emotional "circuit", and their excess or deficit may be reflected in specific clinical symptoms.

1. **Dopamine (DA): the engine of pleasure and motivation**
   - Excess: euphoria, hyperactivity, impulsivity, racing thoughts, grandiosity.
   - Deficit: apathy, anhedonia, sluggishness, loss of interest.

Dopamine is the linchpin of manic states; its excess in the mesolimbic system leads to overstimulation of pleasure and reward. Its descent marks the depressive phases.

2. **Serotonin (5-HT): the emotional thermostat**
   - Relative excess: irritability, anxiety, insomnia.
   - Deficit: sadness, hopelessness, suicidal thoughts, sleep disorders.

Serotonin regulates mood, sleep, and appetite. Serotonin stabilizes emotional sensitivity, but its dysfunction is the hallmark of bipolar depression.

3. **Noradrenaline (NA): energy and alertness**
   - Excess: agitation, insomnia, reactivity, panic attacks.
   - Deficit: fatigue, slowness, cognitive apathy.

Noradrenaline modulates wakefulness and attention. In mania, the "mental volume" increases; in depression it silences him.

4. **GABA (gamma-aminobutyric acid): the emotional brake**
   - Excess: drowsiness, apathy, emotional inhibition.
   - Deficit: anxiety, insomnia, muscle tension, irritability.

GABA is the brain's main inhibitory neurotransmitter. Its deficit is associated with bipolar anxiety and mixed phases.

5. **Glutamate: the thought accelerator**
   - Excess: excessive arousal, insomnia, impulsivity, risk of neurotoxicity.
   - Deficit: cognitive slowness, difficulty concentrating.

Glutamate is involved in memory and learning. Modern research suggests that its dysfunction is key in cyclothymia and affective instability.

6. **Acetylcholine: emotional memory**
   - Excess: emotional hypersensitivity, easy crying, nostalgia, melancholic depression.
   - Deficit: disinterest, confusion, cognitive impairment.

Acetylcholine is linked to REM sleep and affective memories. It is activated during depression, which generates excessive introspection.

7. **Endorphins: the pain buffer**
   - Excess: denial of discomfort, artificial euphoria, reckless behavior.

- Deficit: sensitivity to pain, physical sadness, lack of motivation.

Endorphins are the brain's natural opiates; they balance pleasure and suffering. Its fall is associated with depressive relapses after episodes of stress.

8. **Adrenaline: the vital impulse**
   - Excess: irritability, anxiety attacks, hypervigilance.
   - Deficit: morning fatigue, apathy and difficulty activating the body.

Adrenaline is involved in the stress response. In manic phases, its excess produces autonomic hyperactivation.

9. **Histamine: the molecule of rhythm and awakening**
   - Excess: insomnia, agitation, reactivity to stress.
   - Deficit: drowsiness, lethargy, demotivation.

Histamine regulates the sleep-wake cycle and the release of other neurotransmitters. Some mood stabilizers work by reducing brain histamine.

10. **Melatonin: the guardian of the circadian rhythm**
    - Excess: drowsiness, apathy, daytime desynchronization.
    - Deficit: insomnia, irritability, time confusion.

Melatonin regulates the light inside the body. Its maladjustment is typical in bipolar patients with insomnia or inverted energy cycles.

11. **Oxytocin: the bonding neurotransmitter**
    - Excess: emotional over-involvement, affective dependence.
    - Deficit: isolation, coldness, difficulty in trusting.

Oxytocin connects empathy with mood regulation. Depression and mania can disrupt your release, affecting your ability to relate.

12. **Vasopressin: the regulator of emotional and body balance**
    - Excess: aggressiveness, irritability, impulsivity.
    - Deficit: apathy, demotivation, sleep imbalance.

Vasopressin acts together with cortisol in the stress response and in the regulation of emotional homeostasis.

58.2 Neurochemical Balance as a Therapeutic Art

Treatment for bipolar disorder is largely about restoring harmony between these systems. Mood stabilizers, antipsychotics, and antidepressants act as tuners that correct imbalances between dopamine, serotonin, GABA, and glutamate. But beyond drugs, stability also arises from regular sleep, nutrition, meditation, and psychotherapy, which naturally modulate neurochemical production.

Modern psychiatry recognizes that the bipolar brain is not "defective", but hypersensitive: a system that amplifies life in all its intensities. To understand his chemistry is to understand his poetry: a brain that, when it finds balance, not only thinks, but creates, feels, and transcends with exceptional depth (Figure 57).

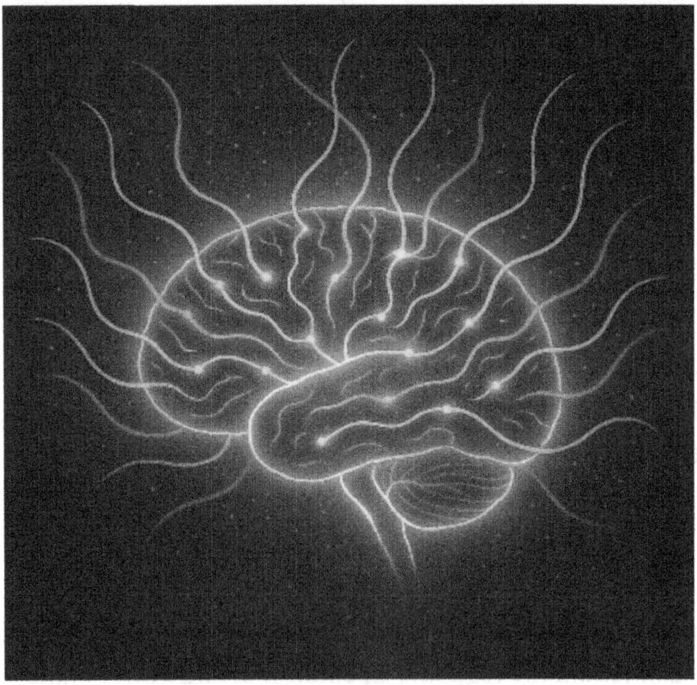

Figure 57. The luminous brain symbolizes neurochemical harmony and balance between the 12 neurotransmitters that regulate the bipolar mind.

CHAPTER 59
Emotional and Neurocognitive Map of Bipolar Disorder

To understand bipolarity is to learn to read an inner map.

59.1 The Brain as an Emotional Territory

Understanding bipolar disorder doesn't just involve studying neurotransmitters or symptoms; It involves drawing a map that connects the inner landscapes of emotion, memory, and consciousness.

The bipolar brain is not chaotic: it is a complex system that tries to self-regulate in the face of extreme sensitivity. Its structure reflects the evolutionary history of the human being: emotion, thought and behavior striving for the same harmony. In the bipolar brain, affective regulation systems are both overactive and vulnerable.

The areas most involved include:

- Amygdala: center of fear, anger, and emotional intensity. In mania, it is hyperactive; In depression, it becomes hypersensitive, which generates disproportionate emotional reactivity.
- Prefrontal cortex: the "conductor" of the brain. It regulates impulses, organizes behavior and modulates emotion. In depressive phases, their activity decreases; in mania, it loses inhibitory control.
- Hippocampus: emotional memory. It is reduced in volume with chronic stress, which affects the ability to learn and regulate affectively.
- Thalamus: point of connection between emotion and cognition. In bipolarity, it transmits emotional messages with excessive intensity.

- Anterior cingulate cortex: Involved in empathy, emotional pain, and decision-making. In bipolar depression, a disconnection with the prefrontal cortex is observed, which explains the difficulty in making rational decisions under states of deep sadness.

The bipolar brain does not "fail"; Vibrates at higher frequencies. It is a brain designed to feel deeply, but it needs to learn to translate that intensity without overflowing.

59.2 Brain Networks: a Desynchronized Symphony

Advances in functional neuroimaging have revealed that bipolar disorder involves alterations in neural networks rather than in isolated regions.

The three most relevant are:

- Default Mode Network: active during introspection and self-referential thinking. In depression, this network dominates, which generates rumination and self-criticism.
- Central Executive Network: Activated during cognitive tasks. In mania, their control is weakened, which favors impulsivity and overestimation of the self.
- Salience network: detects relevant stimuli. In bipolar patients, their hyperactivity explains hypersensitivity to changes in the environment, light, tone of voice or emotional climate.

Treatment seeks to resynchronize these networks through pharmacotherapy, cognitive therapy, stable sleep, and regular habits. In neuroscientific terms, stabilizing mood means restoring rhythm between brain networks that stopped dancing to the same beat.

59.3 The Emotional Map: from Euphoria to Emptiness

From a psychological point of view, the bipolar goes through archetypal emotional states. Each phase represents a point on the affective map:

- Mania: expansion of the ego: The subject feels that he can do anything; the brain releases dopamine in a cascade. There is a sense of creative omnipotence.
- Hypomania: intermediate state, where energy and clarity are combined: Many artists and scientists recount their most productive periods during this phase.
- Depression: Implosion of the self: Life energy is withdrawn, dopamine and serotonin drop, and thinking becomes introspective and pessimistic.
- Mixed phase: the greatest clinical challenge: The mind accelerates but the mood is sunk. Impulsivity is mixed with hopelessness and the risk of suicide is high.
- Euthymia: balance. It is not the absence of emotion, but integration. The brain reaches a point of neurochemical coherence that allows you to think, feel, and act in sync.

This map shows that bipolar disorder is not just a mood disorder, but a disturbance of the rhythm of life. The therapeutic key is to learn to navigate, not to deny the tides.

59.4 The Cognitive Dimension: Thinking, Memory and Judgment

Bipolarity also affects neurocognition, especially in executive functions and memory. Studies show alterations in:

- Processing speed: In manic phases, thinking accelerates; in depression, it slows down.
- Sustained attention: the bipolar mind is easily distracted, because its salience system captures multiple stimuli simultaneously.
- Working memory: Emotional overload interferes with the retention of recent information.
- Judgment and planning: The prefrontal cortex loses control over limbic areas, making it difficult to make coherent decisions in states of high emotional intensity.

Cognitive rehabilitation —along with therapy and structured sleep— helps restore these functions. The goal is not just to "stabilize", but to integrate emotion and cognition to regain a sense of self.

59.5 Consciousness as an Integrating Network

Beyond structures and neurotransmitters, bipolar disorder is an integrative disturbance of consciousness. The bipolar being lives in a continuous stream of amplified internal and external perceptions. His challenge is not to eliminate the intensity, but to transform it into emotional wisdom.

When therapy achieves this integration, the patient does not return to the starting point: a broader, more empathetic and more lucid awareness emerges. The bipolar mind can move from chaos to knowledge. In that transit lies its greatness. It is a system that, once understood, reveals the union between science and soul: the brain as an instrument, and consciousness as its music.

59.6 The Future: Neurocircuits of Hope

Current research explores how deep brain stimulation, artificial intelligence, and genetic biomarkers can predict episodes and tweak personalized treatments.

The neuroemotional map of the future will be interactive: it will integrate biological data, sleep patterns, language and facial expression. The goal will be to prevent, not just treat. But no algorithm can replace human understanding. Because at the heart of the bipolar brain beats something that no machine can measure: the ability to be emotionally reborn.

The emotional and neurocognitive map of bipolar disorder is not a portrait of illness, but an atlas of the human mind at its most intense. Where neuroscience sees networks, poetry sees constellations. And in the center of that electric sky, the bipolar human being learns that balance is not the absence of a storm, but the wisdom of knowing how to navigate it (Figure 58).

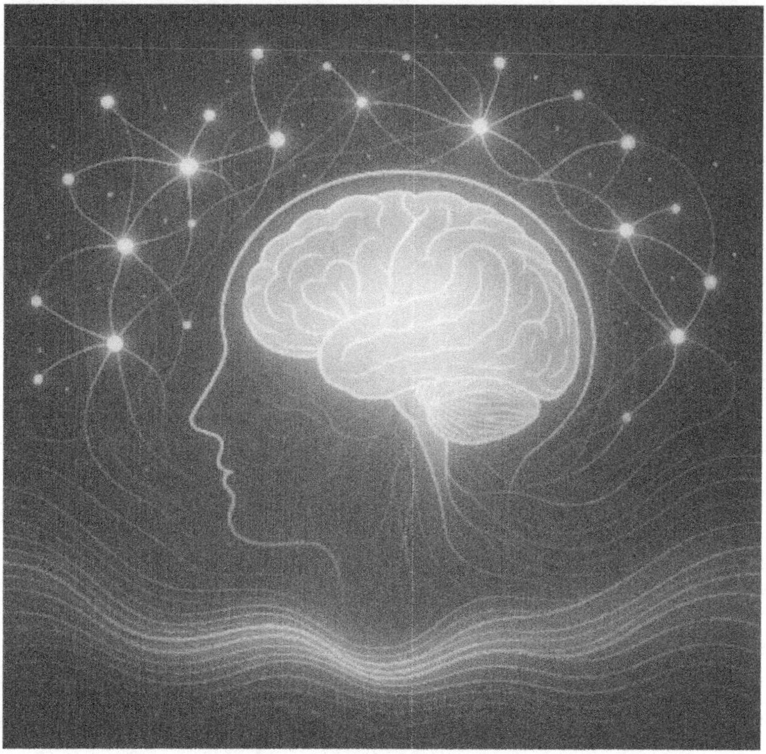

Figure 58. The illuminated brain symbolizes the integration between emotion, thought, and consciousness in the neurocognitive map of bipolar disorder.

CHAPTER 60
Symbolic Gallery of Bipolar Disorder: Painting, Poetry and Cinema

Art does not explain bipolarity: it makes it visible.

60.1 Painting: Emotion Made Color

Art has been, since ancient times, the visible resonance of the invisible states of mind. Bipolarity —that dance between creative euphoria and reflexive melancholy— has inspired some of the greatest geniuses in history.

This chapter does not seek to romanticize illness, but to rescue its symbolic dimension: the ability to transform chemical chaos into meaning, and suffering into beauty.

60.1.1 Vincent van Gogh, the Brush of the Inner Storm

Van Gogh is, perhaps, the universal emblem of bipolar genius. His work is a visual record of the ups and downs of the mood: from the manic energy of The Starry Night, with its vibrant spirals and cosmic rhythm, to the suspended sadness in Wheat Field with Crows.

Modern studies of their correspondence and biography suggest classic symptoms of bipolarity: prolonged insomnia, creative euphoria, irritability, guilt, and periods of depressive exhaustion. His painting became a neurochemical self-portrait: each stroke a synapse, each color an exalted neurotransmitter.

60.1.2 Frida Kahlo, the Body as a Mirror of the Soul

Frida represents the intersection between physical pain and emotional suffering. His painting —intense, symbolic, visceral— shows how the bipolar mind can turn trauma into art.

In paintings such as *The Broken Column* or *The Two Fridas*, the oscillation between vulnerability and strength, between disintegration and the desire for identity, is perceived. Frida sublimated suffering into aesthetics, and in that sublimation she found survival.

60.1.3 Edvard Munch, the Cry of Imbalance

In *The Scream*, Munch paints universal bipolar anxiety: a sky that vibrates, a figure that dissolves into its own emotional echo. His life was marked by periods of isolation, hypersensitivity and panic. Today his work is interpreted as a metaphor for the amplified perception of the bipolar: the world is not seen, one feels with bare nerves (Figure 59).

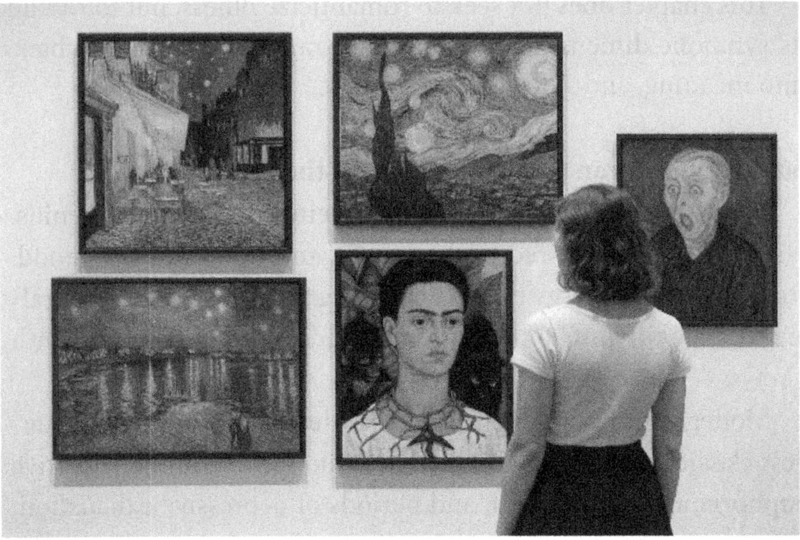

Figure 59. Three souls marked by the emotional intensity of bipolar disorder. Van Gogh, Kahlo and Munch dialogue with a viewer who recognizes in her art a mirror of the fragmented soul.

60.2 Poetry: The Alchemy of Emotion

60.2.1 Sylvia Plath, the Language of the Abyss

Plath transformed depression into a form of poetic lucidity. In *Ariel* he wrote with the voice of the storm: "Silence devours me like a white fire". His work anticipates what neuropsychiatry today calls emotional hyperconnectivity: a sensitivity that captures the invisible nuances of suffering. His poetry shows that the bipolar mind not only suffers; it also perceives with an almost cosmic depth.

61.2.2 Federico García Lorca, the Luminous Tragedy

Lorca combined creative exaltation with existential anguish. In poems such as *Romance sonámbulo*, lyrical euphoria coexists with the shadow of death. His language is bipolar by nature: full of rhythm, desire and melancholy. Lorca embodies the emotional energy that oscillates between creation and sacrifice (Figure 60).

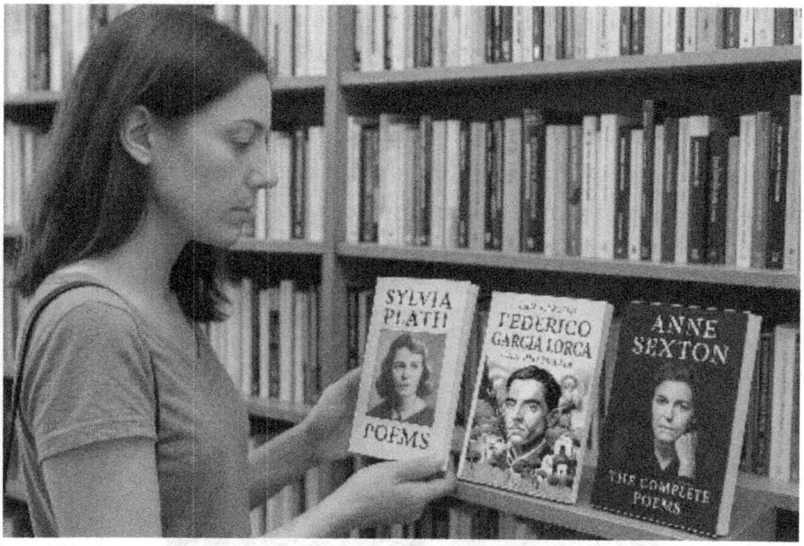

Figure 60. A reader delves into the works of Plath, Lorca and Sexton; three writers whose genius stood out among the chiaroscuro of bipolar disorder and psychic pain.

61.2.3 Anne Sexton, confession as catharsis

Sexton brought poetry to the psychiatrist's office. Her work, born out of pain and therapy, demonstrates that writing is a form of emotional self-regulation. Each poem is an attempt to reintegrate a fractured mind. In it, the word fulfills a function of affective stabilizer.

61.3 Cinema: the Narrative mirror of the Bipolar Mind

61.3.1 *A Beautiful Mind* (2001): The Genius and His Labyrinth

Although focused on schizophrenia, the film reflects the universal dilemma of mental illness: the fine line between creativity and loss of control. John Nash's depiction symbolizes the struggle between reason and perception, so familiar to those who live with bipolarity.

61.3.2 *Silver Linings Playbook* (2012): Love, Chaos and Neurochemistry

Starring Bradley Cooper and Jennifer Lawrence, this film showed bipolar disorder for the first time from an empathetic and everyday perspective. Without stigmas or romanticism, it teaches that love and emotional stability are not opposites, but neurochemical processes in search of harmony (Figure 61).

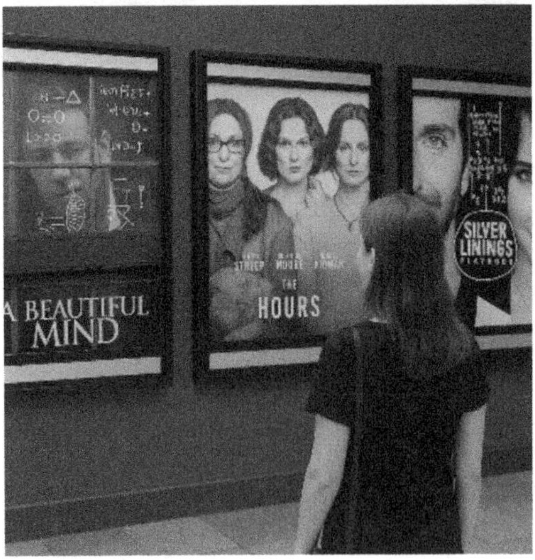

Figure 61. These three films make bipolar disorder visible from different perspectives: genius, pain and love. A woman stops in front of the promotional posters of the three of them, as if recognizing the strength of vulnerability.

61.3.3 *The Hours* (2002): Three Women, one Abyss

Inspired by Virginia Woolf —another figure with probable bipolar disorder— *The Hours* explores how depression is inherited, shared and transformed. The film turns illness into visual language, where water and light symbolize the mind that fluctuates between clarity and dissolution.

61.4 Art as Therapy, Art as a Mirror

Art does not heal on its own, but it heals the invisible. Modern neuroscience shows that creating activates the same dopamine and endorphins circuits as drug treatments. Painting, writing, and music stimulate emotional neuroplasticity and restore the connection between cerebral hemispheres.

In bipolar disorder, art is a form of spontaneous neurotherapy: each creative act reorganizes the wounded brain. Art allows us to name the unnameable. When chemistry overflows, aesthetics picks up the excess and transforms it into meaning. Every stroke, verse or image is an attempt by the soul to tell the brain: "I'm still here".

61.5 Towards an Aesthetics of Stability

In the modern era, the understanding of bipolar art goes beyond the romanticism of tortured genius. Science confirms that creativity is not born from suffering, but from amplified sensitivity that, when channeled, becomes beauty.

A balanced bipolar brain does not lose its intensity: it redirects it. The challenge is not to extinguish the flame, but to learn how to use its light.

Art is not an escape from the bipolar mind: it is its deepest return. In painting, poetry and cinema, the mind finds its mirror and its refuge. Where science sees neurochemistry, art sees meaning. Where the diagnosis speaks of dysfunction, art responds with humanity.

CHAPTER 61
Model B-DNP-21 Applied to Bipolarity

Behind every symptom is a predominant neurochemical system.

61.1 What is the DNP-21 form?

The DNP-21 model (the predominant neurochemical domain of the TWENTY-FIRST century) arises in clinical practice, from the observation of hundreds of patients who did not respond to standard treatments. Based on these cases, recurrent patterns between symptoms and neurochemical profiles were identified, which allowed the design of an initial instrument capable of mapping dysfunctions in a systematic way.

This first instrument gave rise to U-DNP-21 (Universal DNP-21), a tool that generally evaluates all the neurochemical systems involved (DA, 5-HT, NE, GABA, Glutamate, ACh) and orients towards the predominant profile of each patient. Based on their results, the clinician can apply one of the six specific instruments of the model.

The DNP-21model was conceived and developed by Dr. Alexis Gómez González, a clinical psychiatrist with training in neuroscience and advanced psychopharmacology (Cuba and Mexico). The proposal is nourished by years of medical practice, teaching and longitudinal follow-up of thousands of patients. The specialist combined scientific evidence with empathic observation and clinical criteria, as detailed on the website www.dnp21.com

Together with Dr. Alexis Gómez González, the following have contributed to the development of the model:

- Clinical psychologists specialized in symptomatological evaluation.
- Neuropsychologists who collaborated in the design of cognitive sections of the instrument.
- Researchers in neuroimaging and pharmacodynamics.
- Volunteer patients, who contributed their experience, validation and experiential perspective.

61.2 Instrument B-DNP-21–Bipolar Disorder

Bipolar disorder is characterized by alternating episodes of depression and mania or hypomania. On a neurochemical level, this disorder involves oscillating dysregulation in several neurotransmission systems, especially:

- Dopamine (DA): Elevated in manic phases, reduced in depression.
- Noradrenaline (NE): Hyperactive in mania, hypoactive in melancholic depression.
- Glutamate (GLU): Associated with cortical overexcitation in mixed and manic episodes.
- GABA (gamma-aminobutyric acid): Inhibitor affected in excitatory states.
- Serotonin (5-HT): It can be chronically reduced, which affects emotional stability.

61.3 Objective of Questionnaire B-DNP-21

Identifying the predominant neurochemical profile in bipolar patients according to the current phase (depressive, manic or mixed) will allow treatment to be guided:

- B-DNP-21 is composed of 21 items, grouped into 4 domains.
- It assesses symptoms representative of alterations in AD, NE, GLU, and GABA (Table 44).

Table 44. Neurochemical domains of B-DNP-21 and distribution of clinical items

Neurochemical Domain	Neurotransmitter	Items	Example
Domain A	Dopamine	1-5	Fast-paced thinking, grandiosity
Domain B	Noradrenaline	6-10	Excessive energy, impulsivity

Neurochemical Domain	Neurotransmitter	Items	Example
Domain C	Glutamate	11-15	Irritability, flight of ideas, hyperarousal
Domain D	GABA	16-20	Lack of sleep, motor anxiety, disinhibition
Global Symptom	-	21	Combination of mental acceleration + impulsivity

Questionnaire Questions B-DNP-21

Response Scale:

0 = Never.

1 = Sometimes.

2 = Frequent.

3 = Almost always.

A-Dopamine Domain

1. I feel full of great ideas that flow non-stop.
2. I think I have special abilities that others don't understand.
3. My thinking goes faster than I can speak.
4. I feel capable of achieving anything, without limits.
5. I have had reckless or impulsive behaviors without remorse.

B-Noradrenaline Domain

6. I feel full of energy, even without sleep.
7. I talk non-stop and change the subject frequently.
8. I act without thinking about the consequences.
9. I have a hard time sitting still or relaxing.
10. I feel constantly rushed physically and mentally.

C-Glutamate Domain

11. I get irritated easily, even with small things.
12. I have a hard time stopping my thoughts or calming my mind.
13. I have sudden mood swings for no apparent reason.
14. I feel like my mind is going to explode from so much activity.
15. I have quick thoughts that I can't control.

D-GABA Domain

16. I have a hard time falling asleep even when I'm tired.
17. I feel physically restless and tense.
18. I have difficulty curbing my urge to speak or act.
19. I have a hard time organizing my thoughts.
20. I find it difficult to remain silent or calm.

Item 21-Global Assessment

21. My mind and body are in a state of simultaneous acceleration.

Interpretation

- Each domain is scored (maximum 15 points).
- The dominant neurotransmitter is identified based on the highest score.
- The following ranges of affectation can be used:

Scoring	Activation Level
0-5	Mild/Normal
6-10	Moderate
11-15	High/Dysregulated

61.4 DNP-21 Questionnaire–Bipolar Disorder

Instructions: Read each statement and mark with an X the option that best describes how often you have experienced that situation in the last 14 days.

Affirmation	Never (0)	Some-times (1)	Fre-quently (2)	Almost Always (3)
1. I feel full of great ideas that flow non-stop.	☐	☐	☐	☐
2. I think I have special abilities that others don't understand.	☐	☐	☐	☐
3. My thoughtsgoes faster than I can speak.	☐	☐	☐	☐
4. I feel capable of achieving anything, without limits.	☐	☐	☐	☐
5. I have had reckless or impulsive behaviors without remorse.	☐	☐	☐	☐
6. I feel full of energy, even without sleep.	☐	☐	☐	☐
7. I talk non-stop and change oftopic frecuently.	☐	☐	☐	☐
8. I act without thinking about the consequences.	☐	☐	☐	☐
9. I have a hard time sitting still or relaxing.	☐	☐	☐	☐
10. I feel constantly rushed physically and mentally.	☐	☐	☐	☐
11. I get irritated easily, even with small things.	☐	☐	☐	☐
12. I have a hard time stopping my thoughts or calming my mind.	☐	☐	☐	☐

Affirmation	Never (0)	Some-times (1)	Fre-quently (2)	Almost Always (3)
13. I have sudden mood swings for no apparent reason.	☐	☐	☐	☐
14. I feel like my mind is going to explode from so much activity.	☐	☐	☐	☐
15. I have quick thoughts that I can't control.	☐	☐	☐	☐
16. I have a hard time falling asleep even when I'm tired.	☐	☐	☐	☐
17. I feel physically restless and tense.	☐	☐	☐	☐
18. I have difficulty curbing my urge to speak or act.	☐	☐	☐	☐
19. I have a hard time organizing my thoughts.	☐	☐	☐	☐
20. I find it difficult to remain silent or calm.	☐	☐	☐	☐
21. My mind and body are in a state of simultaneous acceleration.	☐	☐	☐	☐

Key to interpretation:

- Items 1-5: dopamine-total: ____________
- Items 6-10: noradrenaline-total: _________
- Items 11-15: glutamato-total: ___________
- Items 16-20: GABA-total: ______________
- Item 21: Global-total evaluation: _________

Nominating neurochemical profile:

____

Suggested therapeutic recommendations:

____

Professional Name:

____

Date: ________________ Signature: ________________

EPILOGUE
Science as a Bridge to Compassion

Every bibliography is, ultimately, a conversation between brains. Scientific knowledge does not replace human experience, it amplifies it. Every study, every neurochemical discovery, every clinical trial on lithium or dopamine has a purpose behind it: to alleviate suffering and restore meaning to existence.

To read about bipolarity is not to study a disease, but to participate in one of the most profound adventures of the TWENTY-FIRST century: to understand how the brain feels, remembers, creates, and loves. Science is the map. Empathy, the path (Figure 62).

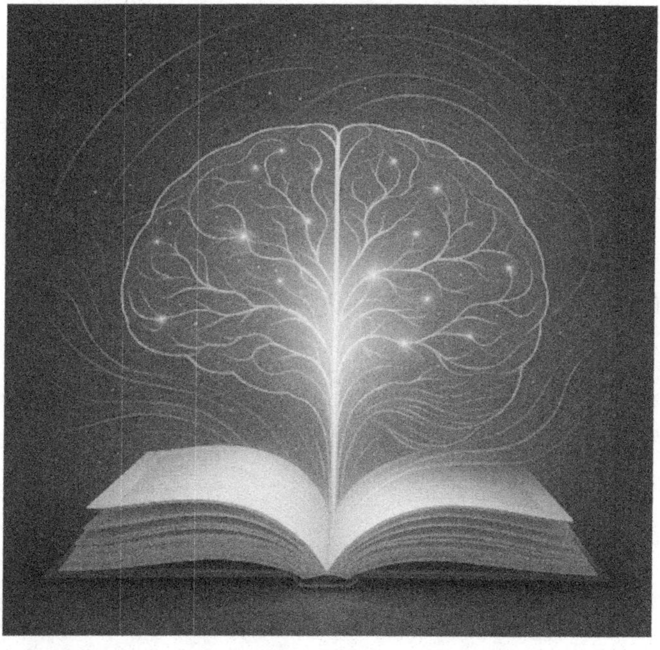

Figure 62. The open brain like a book symbolizes the union between science and wisdom, where knowledge is transformed into human understanding.

ANNOTATED SCIENTIFIC BIBLIOGRAPHY

Science advances when we keep asking.

The understanding of bipolar disorder is constantly evolving. Each decade brings new light on its neurobiology, treatments, and human dimension. This chapter offers an annotated selection of the most relevant works and studies, explained in accessible but scientifically sound language, so that the reader can continue his exploration with criteria and depth.

BIOLOGICAL AND NEUROCHEMICAL FOUNDATIONS

Goodwin, F. K. & Jamison, K. R. (2007). *Manic-Depressive Illness: Bipolar Disorders and Recurrent Depression.* Oxford University Press.

Considered the scientific "bible" on bipolar disorder, its authors –a psychiatrist and a patient-scientist with bipolar disorder– synthesize decades of neurobiological research with clinical observations in the book. She delves into neurotransmitters, genetics and treatment models.

Millan, M. J. & Andrieux, A. (2014). Beyond Monoamines: Emerging Roles of Glutamate and GABA in Mood Disorders. *Trends in Pharmacological Sciences*, 35(1), 36-46.

Key review on the role of glutamate and GABA in emotional regulation. Theoretical basis for the development of future therapies beyond conventional antidepressants.

Nestler, E. J., Hyman, S. E. & Malenka, R. C. (2015). Molecular Neuropharmacology: A Foundation for Clinical *Neuroscience.* McGraw-Hill.

Essential text to understand how psychotropic drugs modulate neurotransmitters and neuronal plasticity. It explains the mechanisms of lithium, valproate, and lamotrigine at the molecular level.

Post, R. M. & Leverich, G. S. (2008). *The Bipolar Spectrum: Diagnostic and Therapeutic Challenges.* American Psychiatric Press.

It introduces the concept of "bipolar spectrum", broadening the vision beyond the classic type I and II model. It includes discussions of cyclothymia and mixed states.

PSYCHOTHERAPY AND INTEGRATIVE APPROACHES

Basco, M. R. & Rush, A. J. (2005). *Cognitive-Behavioral Therapy for Bipolar Disorder.* Guilford Press.

It describes how to adapt cognitive behavioral therapy (CBT) to manic and depressive phases, including strategies for insight and relapse prevention.

Frank, E. et al. (2005). Interpersonal and Social Rhythm Therapy for Bipolar Disorder. *Biological Psychiatry, 57*(5), 496-505.

It describes social rhythm therapy (IPSRT), an intervention based on the regulation of sleep, eating, and social retinas. It combines chronobiology and psychotherapy in a pioneering way.

Linehan, M. M. (2014). *DBT Skills Training Manual.* Guilford Press.

Although created for borderline disorder, dialectical-behavioral therapy (DBT) has shown efficacy in bipolarity, especially in patients with impulsivity and emotional reactivity.

Miklowitz, D. J. (2019). *The Bipolar Disorder Survival Guide: What You and Your Family Need to Know.* Guilford Press.

Practical and empathetic manual that combines clinical evidence with psychoeducational tools. It is a fundamental reference for patients and families.

CULTURAL AND EXISTENTIAL PERSPECTIVES

Jamison, K. R. (1993). *Touched with Fire: Manic-Depressive Illness and the Artistic Temperament.* Free Press.

A work that explores the connection between creativity and bipolarity with sensitivity and historical rigor. It includes analyses of artists, poets, and composers diagnosed with the disorder.

Kleinman, A. (1988). *The Illness Narratives: Suffering, Healing, and the Human Condition.* Basic Books.

Medical anthropologist who analyzes how cultures interpret mental illness. It allows us to understand how bipolarity is experienced and named in different ways in each social context.

Solomon, A. (2012). *Far From the Tree: Parents, Children, and the Search for Identity.* Scribner.

Monumental book on human diversity. Dedicated to families facing neurological, genetic, or psychiatric differences with love and acceptance.

Woolf, V. (1931). *The Waves.* Hogarth Press.

A poetic novel that, although not clinical, reflects with astonishing precision the oscillation of the soul and the fragmented consciousness of bipolarity. Reading it allows a phenomenological understanding of the disorder.

INNOVATIONS, NEUROSCIENCE AND THE FUTURE

Drevets, W. C., Price, J. L. & Furey, M.L. (2008). Brain Structural and Functional Abnormalities in Mood Disorders: Implications for Neurocircuitry Models of Depression and Mania. *Brain Structure and Function, 213*(1-2), 93-118.

A pioneering study in mapping the connectivity between the amygdala, the prefrontal cortex, and the anterior cingulate —the cerebral triangle of mood.

Grande, I., Berk, M., Birmaher, B. & Vieta, E. (2016). Bipolar Disorder. *The Lancet, 387*(10027), 1561-1572.

Scientific review of international reference. It summarizes the current state of knowledge in genetics, pharmacology, and clinical models.

Insel, T. R. (2022). *Healing: Our Path from Mental Illness to Mental Health.* Penguin Press.

The former director of the National Institute of Mental Health of the United States reflects on the errors and promises of the psychiatric system. He proposes a more humane psychiatry, focused on bonding and recovery.

Young, A. H. & Juruena, M. F. (2020). The Neurobiology of Stress and Mood Disorders. *Current Topics in Behavioral Neurosciences, 50,* 1-25.

He describes how stress alters neuronal plasticity and hormonal axes, explaining the biological vulnerability of the bipolar brain.

APPENDICES

Appendix 1. Digital, Educational, and Community Resources

- **International Society for Bipolar Disorders (ISBD)** www.isbd.org: Leading global research and education organization.
- **Depression and Bipolar Support Alliance (DBSA)** www.dbsalliance.org: Support groups, clinical guidelines, and virtual conferences.
- **National Alliance on Mental Illness (NAMI)** www.nami.org: Resources in English and Spanish for patients and families.
- **Telegalenos.com**: Bilingual mental health network with integrative guidance for Spanish speakers.
- **La Fe Clinic.com**: An educational clinical platform that combines psychiatry, psychotherapy, and digital mental health education.

Appendix 2. 100 Frequently Asked Questions in my Consultation

This appendix is born from my own experience as a psychiatrist, from the years I have listened to, accompanied and learned from my patients. Each of these questions does not come from a book, but from a look, from a doubt expressed in the midst of a crisis, from a trembling voice that seeks answers and hope. Through them I have discovered that bipolar disorder is not only a mood disturbance, but a human story written with sensitivity, courage and intensity.

I have gathered here the 100 most frequently asked questions that have been asked by patients, family members and colleagues throughout my clinical practice. Each answer is born from the dialogue between science and experience, between neurobiology and real life. I do not seek to give cold definitions, but to offer clarity, comfort and tools that allow us to understand that bipolarity does not define a person: it invites them to know themselves, to transform themselves and to rediscover balance.

More than a manual, this chapter is a conversation. It's my way of talking to the patient who has just received their diagnosis, to the family member who doesn't know how to help, and to the reader who wants to understand what's going on in their mind or in the mind of someone they love.

I write from the certainty that science, when combined with empathy, truly heals. Because behind every synapse and every neurotransmitter there is a human being with history, with art, with dreams. And if I have learned anything in these years, it is that living with bipolar disorder does not mean being broken: it means having a mind that feels the world with an intensity that, well guided, can become light, creativity and wisdom.

1. **What exactly is bipolar disorder?**

It is a medical condition of the brain that alters the regulation of mood, energy, and behavior. These are not simple "mood swings", but a neurochemical imbalance in neurotransmitters such as dopamine, serotonin, and norepinephrine. These substances fluctuate outside their normal range, an imbalance that causes phases of euphoria (mania or hypomania) and phases of depression. The bipolar brain isn't broken: it's more sensitive and needs to learn how to balance emotion and control.

2. **Can bipolar disorder be cured?**

It has no definitive cure, but it can be completely controlled. With proper treatment, most patients achieve stability, healthy relationships, functionality, and well-being. The goal is functional remission: living well, with minimal or no relapses.

3. **Why is it called "bipolar"?**

Because mood oscillates between two poles: high (mania or hypomania) and low (depression). However, there are intermediate nuances between the two. Today there is more talk of the bipolar spectrum than of a rigid division between two extremes.

4. **Is bipolar disorder hereditary?**

Yes, it has a strong genetic component. If one of the parents suffers from it, the risk to the children is 10%; if both have it, it can reach 30-40%. It is not the exact disease that is inherited, but the biological vulnerability to mood swings.

5. **What causes bipolar disorder?**

It arises from the interaction between genetics, neurochemistry and environmental factors such as stress or trauma. It is a multifactorial disorder in which the brain reacts disproportionately to emotional or biological stimuli.

6. **Is it the same as depression?**

No. Although bipolar depression shares symptoms with major depression, their origin and treatment are different. In bipolar arthritis, antidepressants without stabilizers can cause mania or rapid cycles.

7. **How many types of bipolarity are there?**

There are two main types: type I (with severe manic episodes) and type II (with mild hypomania and deep depression). There are also milder forms such as cyclothymia and the subthreshold bipolar spectrum.

8. How is it diagnosed?

Through a complete psychiatric evaluation, medical history, observation of symptoms and, in some cases, standardized scales. There is no laboratory test to confirm this, although neuroimaging shows characteristic brain patterns.

9. Why is it sometimes confused with depression or ADHD?

Because the depressive phases resemble unipolar depression and hypomania are sometimes confused with the impulsivity of ADHD. The difference is in the presence of recurring cycles of energy and mood.

10. What does it feel like during mania?

Immense energy, racing thoughts, poor sleep, irritability, or euphoria. The patient may feel invincible, overspend or make risky decisions without measuring consequences.

11. And in bipolar depression?

You feel a deep emptiness, slowness, hopelessness and loss of interest. It is not simple sadness, but a chemical disconnection from the pleasure and motivation system.

12. How to distinguish it from normal ups and downs?

Normal changes are brief and proportional. In bipolar, they last for days or weeks and affect daily life. They do not depend on the will, but on neurobiological balance.

13. What neurotransmitters are involved?

Mainly dopamine, serotonin, norepinephrine, GABA and glutamate. Its imbalance alters mood, sleep and perception. Drugs seek to restore harmony between them.

14. How is bipolar disorder treated?

With a combination of medication, psychotherapy, regular sleep, stress management, and family support. It is a comprehensive treatment.

15. What medicines are most commonly used?

Mood stabilizers (lithium, valproate, lamotrigine, carbamazepine), atypical antipsychotics (quetiapine, olanzapine, lurasidone) and, in some cases, antidepressants with caution.

16. Is lithium still useful?

Yes, it is still the "gold standard". It is effective in preventing mania and suicide, although it requires control of levels and kidney function.

17. What side effects can appear?

Although they depend on the drug, some side effects that may appear are weight gain, tremor, drowsiness or metabolic alterations. With regular checks, doses are adjusted to avoid them.

18. What happens if I stop taking medication?

The risk of relapse increases greatly. Abruptly suspending it can cause a new crisis. It should always be done under medical supervision.

19. How long should I take the medicine?

It is usually prolonged. Some patients maintain it for life; others manage to reduce doses after stable years. It is decided on a case-by-case basis.

20. What happens if I am pregnant?

Some medicines are dangerous (such as valproate). The psychiatrist and obstetrician must design a safe plan together. Postpartum is a high-risk period for relapse.

21. What do I do if I have suicidal thoughts?

Seek help immediately. Call emergencies or crisis lines. It is not weakness, it is a treatable symptom. You're never alone.

22. Why is there a higher risk of suicide in patients with bipolarity?

Because of the mixture of hopelessness and impulsivity, especially in mixed phases. Proper treatment drastically reduces that risk.

23. How does it affect sleep?

Sleep is disturbed before mood: sleeping less or more than normal can be the first sign of decompensation.

24. Can stress cause a crisis?

Yes. Stress alters the hormonal axis of the brain and imbalances neurotransmitters. That's why learning to manage stress is essential.

25. Does food have an influence?

Yes. A diet with omega-3s, fruits, vegetables, and magnesium improves emotional balance. Avoiding alcohol, caffeine, and sugar helps control.

26. Can I consume alcohol?

Not recommended. Alcohol alters neurotransmitters and reduces the effect of medications.

27. What about coffee or cigarettes?

Caffeine and nicotine can increase anxiety and insomnia. Caffeine in excess can even induce hypomania.

28. Does exercise help?

Yes. Exercise releases endorphins and increases BDNF, or brain-derived neurotrophic factor, which improves mood and neural plasticity.

29. Why do some patients deny their diagnosis?

During mania, the feeling of well-being prevents recognition of the disease. Education and experience strengthen awareness over time.

30. How can I help a bipolar family member?

With information, patience and empathy. Avoiding arguments during crises, supporting adherence, and recognizing early signs are key.

31. How do you know if a relapse is coming?

Changes in sleep, irritability, appetite, energy, or speech. Detecting it early allows us to act in time.

32. Can you have a normal life?

Yes. With treatment, structure, and support, most lead full lives. Stability is possible.

33. Why are some bipolar people so creative?

Because your brain has a greater connection between emotional and cognitive areas. Channeled correctly, that intensity becomes talent.

34. Can they work?

Yes. Work can be therapeutic if there are stable schedules and understanding of the environment.

35. What is a mixed phase?

When there are symptoms of mania and depression at the same time. It is dangerous and requires urgent attention.

36. What does "fast cycling" mean?

It means having four or more episodes a year. It may be due to hormonal changes, stress, or interruptions in treatment.

37. Do hormones play a role?

Yes. Hormonal changes can destabilize mood, especially in women.

38. How does it present in adolescents?

With irritability, impulsivity or extreme sadness. Early diagnosis improves the prognosis.

39. And in older adults?

Manias are less intense, but depressions are longer. Doses must be adjusted by metabolism.

40. Does therapy work in addition to medication?

Yes. Medication stabilizes chemistry, therapy teaches you to live with it.

41. Which type of therapy is best?

Psychoeducation, cognitive-behavioral, interpersonal and social rhythm therapy.

42. What test should a patient with bipolar disorder have?

Renal, hepatic, thyroid function, and plasma levels of the drug.

43. Does lithium change my personality?

No. It lets you be yourself without going to extremes.

44. Does lithium damage the kidneys?

Only if it is not controlled. With monitoring and good hydration it is safe to take.

45. Why do medications make you feel "flat"?

Because they soften the extremes. It's not a lack of emotion, it's balance.

46. Why may the patient feel "weird" but stable?

Because the brain is getting used to balance. The calm can feel strange after chaos.

47. What happens if the patient misses a dose?

It is recommended not to double the dose and to resume the next dose at your usual time.

48. Does childhood trauma play a role?

Yes. It increases vulnerability to stress and emotional dysregulation.

49. How is it different from borderline disorder?

The bipolar changes by days; the limit, by hours. The origin of bipolar is chemical; that of the limit, emotional and relational.

50. Can someone diagnosed with bipolar disorder study?

Yes, and successfully if there is structure and consistency.

51. Why do some refuse treatment?

Out of fear or denial. Empathy and accompaniment are essential.

52. What can be done if a loved one is manic?

Avoid arguments, reduce stimuli and seek immediate professional help.

53. Does the disorder change over the years?

Yes. The episodes usually become less intense, and the patient learns to self-regulate.

54. Can I have anxiety in addition to bipolar disorder?

Yes, and it is very frequent. It is treated with therapy and emotional regulation strategies.

55. Why are some bipolars so charismatic?

Because in hypomania there is an increase in dopamine, energy and sociability.

56. Does the disorder affect memory?

Yes, during crises. With stability and cognitive exercises, he recovers.

57. What is the difference between hypomania and mania?

Hypomania is mild; mania is severe and requires hospitalization.

58. Can I have stable love relationships?

Yes, as long as there is communication, treatment and understanding.

59. Why do discussions affect me so much?

Because of limbic hypersensitivity. Your brain reacts more intensely.

60. Can I be a good parent?

Yes. With stability and family support, you can be a mindful and caring parent.

61. Why can't I sleep sometimes?

Because your biological clock is still sensitive. The sleep routine is essential.

62. Is bipolarity linked to art?

Yes. Emotional sensitivity stimulates creativity when it is well managed.

63. Can I meditate

Yes, but with caution. Breathing and mindfulness techniques are preferred.

64. Does bipolar disorder have advantages?

Yes, for example: sensitivity, empathy, intuition and creativity. Well channeled, they become fortresses.

65. What is a silent relapse?

Subtle changes in sleep, energy, or mood. Detecting it in time avoids crises.

66. Does spirituality help?

Yes, if it is balanced. It can give purpose and inner peace.

67. How important is the environment?

A lot. Stability needs healthy bonds and firm retinas.

68. How do I deal with the fear of relapse?

With prevention and awareness. Fear can be transformed into wisdom.

69. Why do I feel guilty after a crisis?

Because you regain consciousness. Therapy helps you forgive yourself and learn.

70. How does it affect sexuality?

In mania it increases; in depression it decreases. Talking about it without taboos is part of recovery.

71. Does art or writing help?

Yes. They are forms of emotional self-regulation and stimulate brain plasticity.

72. What is psychoeducation?

Learn about the disease, treatment, and relapses. Psychoeducation empowers the patient and reduces hospitalizations.

73. Can I have a stable job?

Yes, the labor structure can be stabilizing.

74. What if I have addictions?

They complicate the disease. It must be treated in a dual way (addiction and bipolarity together).

75. Do alternative therapies work?

They can complement, not replace. Yoga, meditation, or acupuncture can help under medical guidance.

76. Why do some get irritated instead of euphoric?

Because excess dopamine can be expressed as aggression instead of joy.

77. What does it mean to be in remission?

It means absence of symptoms and normal functional life.

78. What role does the family play?

Family support is essential to prevent relapse and provide emotional stability.

79. Why do some people not respond well to treatment?

Due to genetics, comorbidities or irregular adherence. Pharmacogenetics seeks personalized solutions.

80. What is bipolar neuroplasticity?

The brain's ability to recover after crises. With therapy, sleep, and exercise, the brain is strengthened.

81. Why do the seasons affect me?

Light influences serotonin. Maintaining routines and adequate sun exposure helps.

82. What do I do if new symptoms appear?

Notify the doctor. Acting early prevents serious crises.

83. What is disease awareness?

Recognize that the disorder exists and requires care. Improve with education and time.

84. Why am I so sensitive to rejection?

Because your emotional system reacts with intensity. Therapy helps to reinterpret those experiences.

85. What to do after a hospitalization?

See it as a reset, not a failure. After hospitalization, habits and priorities must be readjusted.

86. Do social networks affect?

Yes. Too much stimulation or comparison can alter mood. Moderation is recommended.

87. Why do I think so much?

Your brain processes faster and deeper. Learning to pause is part of stability.

88. Does music help?

Yes. Regulates dopamine and emotions. Listening to or creating music is therapeutic.

89. Can I travel?

Yes, with planning. Maintain schedules and constant medication.

90. Does it affect self-esteem?

Yes. Relapses can weaken self-esteem, but therapy rebuilds it.

91. What is bipolar grief?

An amplified emotional response to loss. Requires accompaniment.

92. Why do I have a hard time concentrating?

Because of the changes in energy and attention. Training concentration is key.

93. How do I explain my illness to others?

In a simple way: "My brain regulates mood differently, but I am in treatment and stable". Information reduces stigma.

94. What do I do if someone discriminates against me?

Educate calmly or walk away. Your dignity is worth more than the ignorance of others.

95. Can I stop taking medicines?

Only with medical guidance and gradually. Never on his own.

96. Does spirituality help heal?

Yes, when you live with balance. It gives meaning, hope, and purpose.

97. Why is bipolarity associated with genius?

Because controlled hypomania can enhance creativity, but talent arises from balance, not chaos.

98. Can I be proud of my recovery?

Yes, absolutely. Every stable day is a biological and emotional victory.

99. What does it mean to live with bipolar disorder today?

It means understanding that your mind is a powerful instrument that needs tuning, not punishment. It is accepting science and compassion as allies. Living with bipolarity is learning not only to survive extremes, but to create harmony with them.

100. What final message does the psychiatrist give to his patients?

That bipolarity is not a condemnation, but an intense way of living. With knowledge, self-love and treatment, it is transformed into wisdom.

Therapeutic-emotional Glossary

Naming what happens in the mind is
the first step to understanding it.

More than memorizing clinical terms, bipolar disorder requires a language that unites science with experience. In this glossary, each word encloses a map between the chemical and the symbolic, between the symptom and consciousness. To learn its meaning is to learn how to translate the brain into the soul, and vice versa.

Affectivity: The word affectivity comes from the Latin affectus, "to be moved by". It is about the ability to experience emotions, pleasure, sadness or enthusiasm. In bipolar, affectivity is intensified: the world feels stronger, more alive, closer or more distant. To understand affectivity is to understand that emotion is not weakness, but a form of biological intelligence.

Allostasis: The process by which the body achieves stability through change. While homeostasis seeks fixed equilibrium, allostasis dynamically adapts to the environment. In bipolar disorder, this system is stretched to the limit: each mood swing is an attempt by the brain to recalibrate itself. Therapy and self-care reinforce this adaptive capacity.

Anhedonia: Inability to feel pleasure. It reflects a decrease in dopamine and endorphins. In bipolar depression, the world loses color, even what once generated enthusiasm. It is not a lack of will, but an alteration in the mesolimbic circuits of pleasure. Recovery begins when the patient learns that pleasure does not always return suddenly: sometimes it has to be rebuilt with patience.

Self-awareness: The ability to observe one's own emotions, thoughts, and behaviors without judgment. It is the core of cognitive therapy and mindfulness. In bipolar, self-awareness allows us to distinguish between "I" and "my episode", between identity and symptom. Developing it is like learning to read the internal climate of the brain.

Cyclothymia: A mild, chronic form of bipolar disorder, characterized by constant mood fluctuations without major episodes. It represents a low-intensity but persistent chemical oscillation. Clinically, it is a brain that "never shuts down or calms down completely". Cyclothymia teaches that even imbalance can have its own rhythm.

Cortisol: Stress hormone. At normal levels, attention and energy improve. In excess, it deteriorates the hippocampus and alters emotional regulation. In bipolar arthritis, cortisol spikes can trigger relapses, especially after insomnia or conflict. Sleeping, breathing, and meditating are all natural strategies to rebalance your child.

Dysphoria: A state of irritability or generalized discomfort. It's the brain's way of expressing its overload. In bipolarity it usually appears in mixed phases, in which manic energy and depressive sadness coexist. Dysphoria is not anger: it is electrical suffering.

Euthymia: The term euthymia comes from the Greek eu-thymos, "good cheer". It is the state of affective balance where neither euphoria nor depression dominates. This is the therapeutic goal of bipolar treatment. Euthymia does not mean the absence of emotion, but harmony between them. It's the stable melody after the storm.

Homeostasis: The tendency of the body to maintain a constant internal balance. In modern psychiatry, emotional homeostasis involves the ability to maintain a controlled oscillation of neurotransmitters. Bipolar treatment seeks to restore that homeostasis without suppressing vitality.

Insight: Awareness of one's own mental state. To have insight is to know that one is sick without losing one's dignity. In bipolar, insight can fluctuate: during mania it is lost ("I'm not sick"), while in depression it can be painfully excessive ("I know I'm wrong and I can't help it"). Strengthening it is a central therapeutic task.

Neuroplasticity: The brain's ability to reorganize its synaptic connections. It is the biological basis of recovery. Each psychotherapy, physical exercise or new experience stimulates neural plasticity. In the bipolar brain, neuroplasticity allows you to learn from each episode rather than get caught up in it.

Psychoeducation: Pillar of modern treatment. It consists of teaching the patient and their family to recognize symptoms, prevent relapses and manage treatment. It not only informs, but transforms the relationship with the disease. Knowing what's going on in the brain reduces guilt and increases therapeutic collaboration.

Resilience: Ability to recover after the crisis. In neurobiological terms, it is the ability of the nervous system to return to balance after the storm. Resilience is trained with structure, bonds, purpose, and self-compassion. In bipolar disorder, it is not measured by the absence of relapses, but by how quickly you get back on your feet.

Circadian rhythm: Internal biological clock that regulates sleep, body temperature, and hormone secretion. It is the metronome of the mood. In bipolar patients, this rhythm is often out of sync, leading to insomnia, nighttime energy, and daytime fatigue. Regulating sleep is often the first step in stabilizing mood.

Cognitive behavioral therapy (CBT): Addresses the relationship between thought, emotion, and behavior. It teaches the patient to identify cognitive distortions —absolutist, catastrophic, or self-critical ideas— that fuel depressive or impulsive episodes. Its effectiveness is widely demonstrated in the treatment of bipolar disorder.

Interpersonal and social rhythm therapy: Model developed by Ellen Frank et al. It integrates psychotherapy with the regulation of biological routines (schedules, sleep, food). It helps the patient stabilize the social rhythms that influence the internal clock. Its clinical motto could be: order life to order the brain.

Drug therapy: Not only a medical tool, but a form of chemical engineering of balance. Lithium, anticonvulsants, and antipsychotics modulate neuronal communication. The success of treatment depends on both the drug and the patient-doctor alliance, which decides when to adjust and when to wait.

Mixed disorder: Phase where symptoms of mania and depression coexist. It is the most dangerous and complex state of the bipolar spectrum. The brain is overloaded with energy, but emotionally desperate. It requires immediate medical attention. It represents the paradox of the mind speeding up as it sinks.

Therapeutic will: It is the profound decision to actively participate in recovery. It goes beyond taking medication: it involves taking emotional responsibility, cultivating healthy habits, and recognizing limits without losing hope. In bipolarity, the therapeutic will turns the diagnosis into a destiny overcome.

The therapeutic-emotional glossary is, at its core, a compass. It allows the complexity of clinical language to be translated into the language of human experience. Each word described here is a tool, a bridge between medical knowledge and the emotional wisdom that lives in every patient who decides to heal.

Telegalenos a gabacha quitá Collection

A Compassionate, Scientific, and Practical Guide to Facing the Challenges of the Mind and Soul

The *Telegalenos a gabacha quitá* Collection was born with a clear mission: to accompany, inform and relieve. Each volume is dedicated to a specific mental health condition, and becomes an intimate conversation between the reader and the psychiatrist. With accessible yet rigorously scientific language, the books address symptoms, causes, treatments, myths, and possibilities for recovery.

More than just manuals, these texts integrate the perspective of medical aikido, a humanistic and dynamic approach to transforming emotional suffering into inner strength. In addition, each book includes up-to-date directories of sources of help in Mexico, Spain, and the United States, and offers real bridges to treatment and community accompaniment.

If you found this book on bipolarity useful or revealing, we invite you to discover the other titles in the collection:

Insomnia

"Sleeping is not giving up, it is an act of health". Chronic insomnia is a silent epidemic. Here you will discover the neurobiological causes, dysfunctional beliefs that perpetuate it, and the most effective strategies for regaining sleep, such as cognitive behavioral therapy for insomnia, sleep hygiene, body relaxation techniques, and pharmacological alternatives when necessary.

Anxiety

"When the alarm system never goes off". This book guides you through the different forms of anxiety —generalized, panic, phobic, social— and their effects on body and mind. It offers practical tools such as somatic breathing, graded exposures, mindfulness, and pharmacotherapy. With a medical aikido approach, you will learn how to transform anxiety into channeled life energy and seek timely help when fear becomes chronic.

ADHD

"It's not a lack of will, it's a brain that works differently". An essential book for parents, diagnosed adults and professionals. It presents current scientific studies, pharmacological options (such as methylphenidate and atomoxetine), school accommodations, and behavioral therapies. In addition, it explores how to channel the energy of Attention Deficit Hyperactivity Disorder (ADHD) into creativity, compassionate organization, and self-understanding through mental aikido techniques.

Dementia

"Memory fades, but love remains". A warm and scientific guide for those living with dementia and their caregivers. The book addresses Alzheimer's, frontotemporal dementia, vascular dementia and Lewy bodies with diagnostic criteria, non-pharmacological strategies, legal guidance, behavior management and emotional containment of the caregiver. Medical aikido proposes a way to accompany with respect, dignity and deep connection.

Addiction

"The void is not filled with substances, but with meaning". This book explores the neurobiological basis of addiction, the cycle of compulsion, the social and psychological factors involved, as well as models of recovery: from medical treatment to harm reduction approaches, 12-step groups, motivational therapy, and secular spirituality. The author offers keys to get out of stigma and punishment, embracing self-compassion and personal agency.

Schizophrenia

"Seeing another reality is not madness, it is suffering on another frequency". Clinically sensitive and non-sensational, this book explains the positive and negative symptoms, the evolution of the disorder, current drug treatments, psychosocial approaches, and how support networks can make a difference. Through medical aikido, schizophrenia is approached as a struggle for internal coherence, where it is possible to accompany without fear and with meaning.

Depression

"The body is silent about what the soul cannot express". It explores the neurochemical mechanisms, emotional wounds, and social circumstances that can lead to a depressive state. This book offers everything from diagnostic criteria to integrative interventions: pharmacological, psychotherapeutic, somatic and spiritual. It includes emotional regulation techniques, help resources in three countries and a special chapter on how to accompany those who suffer without falling into judgment or despair.

Autism

This book is not about "correcting" an autistic child... try to understand it. Every autistic mind deserves a world that understands it. It is a warm, clear, and hope-filled guide for families seeking real answers, professionals who want to learn, and autistic adults who deserve to be heard. It's a journey into the most beautiful thing about neurodevelopment: authenticity. It is not a manual. It is not a diagnosis. It's a hug.

Why choose this collection?

- Because it is written by a clinical psychiatrist with experience in consultation, emergencies and therapy.

- Because it is based on up-to-date scientific studies and international guidelines.
- Because it has an understandable language, without losing scientific precision.
- Because it includes non-pharmacological approaches, integrative medicine, and spirituality.
- Because it integrates the model of medical aikido: anticipate, contain, transform.
- Because it provides real help resources in three countries: Mexico, Spain, and the United States.
- Because it was designed for patients, family members and professionals.

Explore, understand and accompany. *Telegalenos a gabacha quitá* is more than a collection of books: it is a community of knowledge, compassion, and possibility.

Made in the USA
Monee, IL
04 November 2026

67378010R00236